PEDIATRIC DIFFERENTIAL DIAGNOSIS

A Problem-Oriented Approach

Second Edition

Pediatric Differential Diagnosis

A Problem-Oriented Approach

Second Edition

Stephen H. Sheldon, D.O.
*Director, Division of Educational Research
and Systems Development
Department of Pediatrics
Mount Sinai Hospital Medical Center
Assistant Professor, Pediatrics and Preventive Medicine
Rush Medical College
Chicago, Illinois*

Howard B. Levy, M.D.
*Chairman, Department of Pediatrics
Mount Sinai Hospital Medical Center
Associate Professor of Pediatrics
Rush Medical College
Chicago, Illinois*

Raven Press ■ New York

Raven Press, 1140 Avenue of the Americas, New York, New York 10036

© 1985 by Raven Press Books, Ltd. All rights reserved. This book is protected by copyright. No part of it may be reproduced, stored in a retrieval system, or transmitted, in any form or by any means, electronic, mechanical, photocopying, recording, or otherwise, without the prior written permission of the publisher.

Made in the United States of America

International Standard Book Number 0-88167-112-6

Library of Congress Cataloging in Publication Data

Sheldon, Stephen H.
   Pediatric differential diagnosis.

   Includes bibliographies and index.
   1. Children—Diseases—Diagnosis.   2. Diagnosis,
Differential.   I. Levy, Howard B.   II. Title.
[DNLM: 1. Diagnosis, Differential—in infancy &
childhood.   WS 141 S544p]
RJ50.S53   1985   618.92′0075   85-42891
ISBN 0-88167-112-6

   Great care has been taken to maintain the accuracy of the information contained in the volume. However, Raven Press cannot be held responsible for errors or for any consequences arising from the use of the information contained herein.

Preface

Children do not present to the health care provider with complaints of a disease. They come with signs and symptoms related to specific disorders. It is said, "If you never think of it, you'll never diagnose it." Without the establishment of an appropriate differential diagnosis, the actual diagnosis never may be established.

The arrival at a diagnosis is not a mystical journey. Physicians are not anointed with a power to diagnose. At all levels of patient contact, the physician is constantly developing hypotheses about what could be wrong, testing the hypotheses with questions and clinical skills, ordering the hypothesis set, and then reordering it according to information received. The cornerstone of a physician's development in reaching a diagnosis is the adequacy and completeness of the differential diagnosis. Appropriate hypothesis generation, deductive reasoning from the analysis of historical data, and appropriate interpretation of physical findings is the basis for arriving at diagnostic closure. The diagnosis should be suspected well before any laboratory tests are ordered.

This manual has been written to assist medical students, residents, pediatricians, nurses, and family practitioners in developing appropriate hypotheses and a differential diagnosis. It is not a "cookbook guide" to diagnosis and management. It is not a textbook of pediatrics, inclusive of all aspects of patient care. Rather, it is a tool for assisting thought processes. Vital clinical points differentiating one disease entity from another are listed. It is small, so the busy house officer, student, nurse, or practitioner may easily carry it in a coat or jacket pocket.

Many chapters of this 2nd edition have been revised and expanded and six chapters have been added. Also new to this edition are the diagnostic charts appearing at the end of many chapters. These charts should provide rapid, at-a-glance comparison of the major signs and symptoms related to specific disease processes. The greatest difficulty one encounters when using these charts is answering the question: Is this sign- or symptom-specific for this disease? The answer in most cases is: It depends. The presence or absence of a specific sign or symptom in any disease process is dependent on many factors. It is the *pattern* of signs and/or symptoms that leads to the suspected diagnosis.

We hope this text will provide a valuable tool for the busy practitioner to better assess and care for sick children.

Stephen H. Sheldon
Howard B. Levy

Preface to the First Edition

The primary goal of pediatric residency training is to provide an educational environment that encourages the acquisition of knowledge, the understanding of basic principles, and the development of professional skills. A major aspect of these professional skills is the ability to make a differential diagnosis.

Increased diagnostic skill results initially from intuitive deduction from the analysis of historical data and the appropriate interpretation of physical findings. Accurate direction of diagnostic pursuit is the consequence of an instinctive response resulting from the ability to assimilate basic principles, acquired knowledge, and past experiences.

The differential diagnosis is the cornerstone of the deductive reasoning process in clinical medicine. Without considering the various etiologies for a specific presenting sign or symptom, a correct diagnosis may never be established. This manual should therefore be utilized to organize thought processes. It is not a "cookbook of medicine."

This handbook has been prepared to assist the busy pediatric house officer in establishing a useful differential diagnosis. It will also be of use to medical students and interns during their rotations through pediatric services. The encyclopedic format is not inclusive, but provides a valuable tool highlighting significant problems that continually confront the pediatrician.

Joseph R. Christian, M.D.
Professor and Chairman
Department of Pediatrics
Rush Medical College

Acknowledgments

Many thanks are in order. First, to the house staff of the Rush Medical College Integrated Pediatric Residency Program and the students of Rush Medical College, whose inquisitiveness and enthusiasm inspired this volume. Second, to Peter Noronha, M.D., Director of Student and Resident Programs in the Department of Pediatrics of Mount Sinai Hospital Medical Center, whose constant input and encouragement of students, residents and attending staff permits arrival at appropriate differential diagnoses. Finally, to the staff of Raven Press, whose hard work, confidence, constant reviews, criticisms, and patience made this endeavor possible.

Contents

Authors' Note

A graphic representation of the differential diagnosis of various presenting problems follows many chapters. Numerical interpretation of the charts is as follows:

0 = The sign or symptom is variable and its presence or absence is not helpful in the diagnosis (e.g., may be present in < 5% of patients with the diagnosis).

1 = The sign or symptom is occasionally present. It may be helpful in the diagnosis (e.g., may be present in < 15% of patients with the diagnosis).

2 = The sign or symptom is often present and helpful in the diagnosis (e.g., may be present in < 50% of patients with the diagnosis).

3 = The sign or symptom is statistically predictable for the diagnosis (e.g., may be present in > 50% of patients with the diagnosis).

4 = The sign or symptom is routinely present and often considered as implicit in the diagnosis (e.g., may be present in > 85% of patients with the diagnosis).

(4) = The sign or symptom is often implicitly *absent* in the diagnosis and is considered as a *pertinent negative* finding.

* = The sign or symptom is not necessarily part of the disease process, but it may be a frequent indication of sequelae.

1–4 (e.g.) = The sign or symptom is extremely variable in presentation. It may or may not be present and may or may not be significant in the diagnosis. The significance may be affected by the presence of other associated signs or symptoms.

Every attempt has been made to represent accurately the symptoms of each disease process. It must be remembered, however, that *disease presentation varies with each patient.* The variation may be considerable. Therefore, each sign or symptom should be evaluated within the context of each patient and situation.

Abdominal Masses

The palpation of an abdominal mass is usually a cause of great concern to physicians treating children. The etiology of the mass may range from benign, nonpathological conditions to extremely malignant, life-threatening tumors. When a mass is palpated, its size, consistency, configuration, position, mobility, and tenderness should be delineated. The presence of additional systemic signs should be investigated. Minimal manipulation of the mass should be permitted once it is sufficiently demonstrated and documented. Ultrasonography, computed tomography, upright and supine plain radiographs, and intravenous pyelography may be utilized to assist in the diagnosis.

Fecal Mass	A fecal mass may be palpated in children who are constipated and have large amounts of retained stool in the colon. The mass may be located anywhere along the course of the large bowel. It may be irregular and freely movable, but is rarely tender. Pain may or may not be present. The mass may feel firm and suggest an intraabdominal neoplasm. With time, the fecal mass will move or resolve after stooling.
Hydro-nephrosis	Hydronephrosis may present as a palpable abdominal mass or may be discovered during investigation of a urinary tract infection or trauma to the kidney. In the younger child, symptoms may appear as a localized urinary tract infection or a systemic infection. Vomiting, septicemia, failure to thrive, and a palpable abdominal mass should alert the clinician to the possible presence of hydronephrosis. In

Hydro-nephrosis (cont'd)	older children, the symptoms are usually referable to the gastrointestinal tract. Symptoms may be nonspecific. Abdominal or flank pain may be present. Gross or microscopic hematuria may occur with minimal trauma. Transillumination may reveal the nature of the mass. Sonography, intravenous pyelography, voiding cystourethrography, retrograde pyelography, and/or cystoscopy may assist in making the diagnosis.
Megaureter	A palpable abdominal mass may or may not be present. Megaureter may be first diagnosed on intravenous pyelography done as part of a work-up for other urinary tract abnormalities or abdominal pain. It is usually not an isolated finding, and further investigation into the cause of the enlargement of the ureter is essential.
Polycystic Kidneys	Two types of polycystic kidney disease are identified. The infantile form (autosomal recessive) is characterized by oligohydramnios, abdominal distention, palpable abdominal or flank masses, respiratory distress, and/or congestive heart failure. Hypertension is common. Gross or microscopic hematuria may occur. Children who survive the neonatal period usually develop hepatic fibrosis, portal hypertension, and progressive renal failure. In the adult type of polycystic kidney disease (autosomal dominant), symptoms may be absent in childhood. Hypertension, intermittent hematuria, and slowly progressive renal failure may occur.
Intraabdominal Organs	Intraabdominal organs may normally be palpated. They may be difficult to distinguish from an abdominal mass. Their palpation may

Intraabdomi-nal Organs (cont'd)	or may not indicate enlargement or abnormal position within the abdomen.
Wilm's Tumor	Children with Wilm's tumor usually present with a palpable abdominal mass. It is not unusual for the parent to discover the mass or complain of difficulty in pinning or taping the child's diapers. Abdominal distention may be present, along with variable abdominal discomfort. Vomiting and/or fever may occur. The mass is usually unilateral, rarely crosses the midline, and is described as smooth and firm. Hypertension may be present. Gross hematuria occurs in approximately 25% of the patients. Hepatomegaly may indicate metastasis to the liver.
Neuroblastoma	Neuroblastoma often presents as an intraabdominal mass, but the presentation depends on the location of the primary tumor, the age of the child, and the presence of metastasis. The mass is usually firm and irregular and often crosses the midline. Rapid enlargement of the mass may suggest hemorrhage into the tumor with resultant anemia and pallor. The presence of a cervical mass may indicate the location of the primary tumor or metastasis. Unilateral proptosis, ecchymosis, and periorbital swelling may indicate metastasis and may be the presenting symptoms. Occasionally, hypertension is present. Fever, bone pain, weight loss, pancytopenia, and abnormal involuntary muscular movements usually indicate extensive disease.
Pancreatic Pseudocyst	Pseudocyst of the pancreas may follow blunt abdominal trauma. Tenderness may be present. The mass tends to be firm and globular. Abdominal pain, anorexia, and vomiting may also be present.

| Other Causes of Intraabdominal Masses | Lymphoma, rhabdomyosarcoma, pyloric stenosis, inflammatory bowel disease, intussusception, choledocal cyst, abdominal aorta, hydrops of the gall bladder, bowel duplication, anterior meningomyelocele, urachal cyst, ovarian cysts and tumors, teratomas, and pregnancy. |

Abdominal Pain

Abdominal pain in the infant is difficult to assess. The history is usually secondhand information. The infant cannot communicate that pain is present. The parents may state that "the baby appears to be having pain." The cry may be "different," feedings may be refused, activity patterns disrupted, or the parent may "just know something is wrong."

The physician must then search for other aspects in the history that may yield a clue. Are there any associated illnesses? How long has the baby been acting like this? Exactly when did the pain start? Has there been a new food added to the diet? Does the pain appear constant or intermittent? Is the baby coughing? Is there any vomiting? Are the baby's stools normal? Is the baby eating and urinating normally? Probably the most important question to ask is: Exactly how is the baby being fed?

In older children, it is important to determine the onset, location, and character of the pain, as well as the presence or absence of associated symptoms and signs.

Abdominal pain is a frequent symptom in times of stress. A careful psychosocial history must be obtained.

Colic	This is the most common cause of abdominal pain in infancy, though the exact etiology is unknown. The child is otherwise well. The pain is paroxysmal and at times difficult to differentiate from the pain of intussusception. The baby may pass large amounts of flatus and burp frequently. Colic most frequently occurs in the firstborn child. It often reflects parental anxiety. Feeding patterns must be investigated.

Gastroenteritis	The etiology may be infectious (bacterial, viral or parasitic), toxic, or irritative. Associated symptoms may be diarrhea, vomiting, hematochezia, fever, and refusal of feedings. Other family members may be affected. Food intolerance may also cause abdominal pain with gastroenteritis. Check stool for bacteria, ova, parasites, blood, pH, and reducing substances.
Constipation	The character of the stool tends to be more important than its frequency. The stools are very hard, dry, and frequently described as "marbles." The pain is described as an ache, usually diffuse and constant. The child is usually not ill. Straining to move the bowels does not mean constipation.
Appendicitis	Physical findings are extremely variable and classic findings are usually absent. The location and character of the pain vary with the position of the appendix. At onset, the pain may be diffuse or periumbilical, later localizing to the right lower quadrant. The pain is usually continuous but is occasionally intermittent. The patient's appetite is usually not altered early in the disease process. Vomiting is usually present. The temperature, as well as the white blood cell count, may be elevated. Point tenderness in the right lower quadrant suggests appendicitis; however, this is variable, depending on the location of the appendix. Sudden cessation of the pain in a sick child may indicate perforation. A barium enema that shows filling of the appendix may exclude appendicitis. The infection, however, may be localized at the tip of the appendix, resulting in appendiceal filling, rendering this radiographic finding unreliable. If the appendix does not fill, appendicitis may or may not be

Appendicitis (cont'd)	present. Visualization of a fecalith in the appendix supports the diagnosis of appendicitis.
Mesenteric Lympha-denitis	History, physical findings, and laboratory examinations may be identical to those in appendicitis. The appendix can usually be visualized with a barium enema. Stools should be cultured for routine enteric pathogens (*E. coli, Salmonella,* and *Shigella*), as well as for less common organisms such as *Yersinia Enterocolitica* and *Campylobacter* species.
Intussusception	Abrupt onset, paroxysmal pain (with the painful episode usually followed by lethargy), bloody stools ("currant jelly"), and a palpable abdominal mass or a mass palpated on rectal examination in a sick-looking child support this diagnosis. Early in the course of intussusception, currant jelly stools are usually absent. The pain may be preceded by a large normal stool. Blood in the feces most often signifies longer standing disease. A mass may be palpated in the right lower quadrant. Barium enema is used for both diagnosis and reduction. If barium enema fails to reduce the intussusception, surgical reduction is necessary.
Ulcerative Colitis	The pain is usually colicky and not extremely severe; it may be made worse by food. Tenesmus is commonly present. Bloody diarrhea with pus and mucus is frequently the first symptom. Anorexia, nausea, and vomiting are later symptoms. Hypochromic microcytic anemia may be present. Malabsorption of fat may also be present; D-xylose absorption test may be abnormal. Barium enema or endoscopy may be diagnostic. Backwash ileitis may occur.

Crohn's Disease	The pain is crampy and exacerbated by eating. It is usually more severe than the pain of ulcerative colitis. Defecation yields some relief. The pain may be periumbilical or localized. Frequent loose stools are characteristic, but bloody mucopurulent stools are less common than in ulcerative colitis. Hypoalbuminemia is invariably present. Malnutrition is commonly present. Rectal involvement may be present. Other extraintestinal manifestations are peripheral edema, clubbing of digits, stomatitis, arthritis, and erythema nodosum. Endoscopy, biopsy, and upper and lower gastrointestinal series may be diagnostic.
Hepatitis	The pain is nonspecific. It may be localized to the right upper quadrant. Anorexia, fatty food intolerance, history of drug abuse, history of contact with an infected person, jaundice, hepatomegaly, joint pain, and elevated transaminase levels support the diagnosis. Serology may be diagnostic, but negative serological tests do not rule out the diagnosis.
Urinary Tract Infection	Nonspecific abdominal pain localized to the suprapubic or flank regions, dysuria, frequency, urgency, incontinence, hematuria, fever, and pyuria support the diagnosis of urinary tract infection. Culture of the urine is imperative.
Other Etiologies	Volvulus, strangulated or incarcerated hernia, pyloric stenosis or spasm, perforation, annular pancreas, Meckel's diverticulitis, diabetes mellitus, testicular or ovarian torsion, ovarian cysts, abdominal epilepsy, sickle cell crisis, plumbism, infectious mononucleosis, porphyria, gall bladder disease, primary peritonitis, pancreatitis, mumps, cystic fibrosis, Henoch-Schönlein purpura, hemolytic-uremic syndrome, hydronephrosis, and pneumonia.

Cause of Abdominal Pain	Location Diffuse	Character Constant	Vomiting	Diarrhea	Anorexia	Constipation	Hematochezia	Anemia	Jaundice	Mass	Perirectal Lesions	Fever	Associated with Food	Relieved with Food	Localized	Paroxysmal
Colic	3	0	0	0	0	0	0	0	0	0	0	0	0	0	0	4
Acute gastroenteritis	3	0	3	4	2	0	1	0	0	0	0	3	0	0	0	0
Constipation	4	2	0	0	0	4	2	0	0	1	2	0	0	0	0	2
Appendicitis	1–4	4	3	0	1–4	1	0	0	0	0	0	4	0	0	1–4	0
Mesenteril lymphadenitis	1–4	4	3	0	1–4	1	0	0	0	0	0	3	0	0	1–4	0
Intussusception	0	0–2	1	0	1–3	0	0	0	0	4	0	1	0	0	4	4
Ulcerative colitis	3	0	3	3	3	0	3	2	0	1	0	2	3	0	0	0
Crohn's disease	1–4	0	0	3	0	0	2	3	0	0	3	2	3	0	2–4	0
Hepatitis	3	3	2	1	4	3	0	0	4	0	0	3	0	0	3	0
UTI	0	4	0	0	0	0	0	0	0	0	0	3	0	0	2	0
Pneumonia	2	3	1	0	1	0	0	0	0	0	0	1	0	0	2	4
Food intolerance	4	1	1	4	1	0	2	0	0	0	0	2	4	0	0	0
Toxin ingestion	4	1–4	1	3	2	0	0	0	0–4	0	0	2	0	0	0	0
Peptic ulcer	2	3	3	0	0	0	2	2	0	0	0	1	3	3	3	4

Abdominal Trauma (Blunt)

Injury to the abdominal viscera should be considered in any child with abdominal trauma. Other injury may be absent. The apparent degree of trauma may be minimal. The exact location of the injury may yield insight into specific organ involvement.

The most important aspect of the initial evaluation is the determination of the presence or absence of an abdominal catastrophe. Once catastrophe is ruled out, "tincture of time" may be the only treatment necessary.

Liver Laceration	This is one of the most urgent intraabdominal injuries encountered after blunt trauma to the right side of the abdomen or chest. The patient is usually in shock. The pain is severe, is usually located in the right upper quadrant, and is increased by respiratory efforts. The patient is anxious but usually lies motionless since motion also increases the pain. There may be referred pain to the right shoulder. There are usually a falling hematocrit, hypotension, pallor, and tachycardia. The mortality rate is quoted as being as high as 40%.
Splenic Laceration	The spleen is the intraabdominal organ most commonly injured in abdominal trauma. Shock may ensue rapidly or rupture may be delayed for a few hours or days. Splenic rupture should be suspected if the trauma was to the left side of the abdomen or chest. Kehr sign (left shoulder pain in the supine position) may be present. Other signs of abdominal catastrophe (shock, hypotension, falling hematocrit, et cetera) are usually present.

Kidney	The pain of a ruptured kidney is localized to the lumbar region. Hematuria is often present. An intravenous pyelogram is ordinarily indicated in patients with significant abdominal trauma.
Pancreas	Signs and symptoms of pancreatic injury may not become immediately apparent. The trauma may be relatively mild and the patient may be symptomless after the injury. A few weeks after the injury, symptoms of a pancreatic pseudocyst may appear. Periumbilical or epigastric abdominal pain, back pain, palpable abdominal mass, and elevated amylase levels suggest pseudocyst formation.
Gastrointestinal Tract and Lower Urinary Tract	Injury to solid viscera is more common than to hollow viscera. Perforation or hematoma can occur after blunt trauma. The signs and symptoms are those of an acute abdomen. Free air may be present under the diaphragm. If a hematoma of the intestinal wall is present, signs and symptoms of intestinal obstruction will occur.

Anemia

Anemia may be acute or chronic. The signs and symptoms manifested depend on the etiology of the anemia, the length of time the anemia has been present, the degree of anemia, the presence of other contributing conditions, and the patient's age.

The history can provide a great deal of information and point toward a specific etiology. Specific questions should be asked regarding fatigue, pallor, blood loss, trauma, and drugs. Neonatal and family history will provide information regarding genetically determined etiologies. Nutritional and socioeconomic factors play an important role in the etiology of anemia.

Important objective information, such as the presence of pallor, tachycardia, jaundice, petechiae, ecchymosis, trauma, tumors, hepatomegaly, and splenomegaly, should be noted. The complete blood cell count, platelet count, reticulocyte count, hemoglobin electrophoresis (patient's and parent's), glucose-6-phosphate dehydrogenase (G-6-PD) levels, blood type, Coombs' test, and bone marrow studies should be considered in the evaluation.

If a blood transfusion is necessary, always draw all specimens for laboratory studies *before* transfusion.

Anemia can be divided into five basic categories: blood loss, nutritional, hemolytic, defective erythropoiesis, and infectious. The differential diagnosis will be discussed according to these categories.

Blood Loss	There are two types of anemia secondary to blood loss: acute and chronic. Both may be caused by overt or covert bleeding. Acute

Blood Loss (cont'd)	anemia will show a rapid decrease in the hemoglobin and hematocrit, with normochromic-normocytic red cell indices. Symptoms appear early and at higher hemoglobin levels. Chronic blood loss will appear as a hypochromic-microcytic anemia as long as no other factors are involved. Lower hemoglobin levels may be reached before symptoms appear.
Placental/ umbilical bleeding	Newborn. Signs of prenatal or natal bleeding. Gross umbilical hemorrhage.
Feto-fetal transfusion	Twins.
Hemorrhagic disease of newborn	Onset between 24 and 120 hours of age. Signs and symptoms of a coagulation defect are petechiae, ecchymosis, purpura, and overt bleeding. There is a marked deficiency in the vitamin K-dependent clotting factors prothrombin and factors VII, IX, and X.
Cephalo-hematoma	Occipital swelling. Does not cross the midline.
Epistaxis	Anterior or posterior nasal bleeding.
Gastrointes-tinal bleeding	Esophageal varices, hiatal hernia, drugs, parasites, hemangiomas, Meckel's diverticulum, ulcerative colitis, polyps, and Henoch-Schönlein purpura.
Urinary tract bleeding	Hemorrhagic cystitis, foreign body, drugs, and stones.
Trauma	
Blood dyscrasias	Coagulation disorders and malignancies.
Nutritional	This is the most common cause of anemia after 9 months of age. The diet may be deficient in iron and protein, with an excess of carbohydrate and milk products. Prolonged breast

Nutritional (cont'd)	feeding may also result in nutritional anemia. The hemoglobin levels may be as low as 3 g percent, with few symptoms. Exact dietary history is imperative. The red blood cell indices are usually hypochromic and microcytic; however, megaloblastic anemias may occur.
Anemia of prematurity	Initially normochromic-normocytic, later hypochromic-microcytic.
Prolonged breast feeding	
Malabsorption syndrome	Malabsorption of iron, malabsorption of fat-soluble vitamins, malabsorption of protein, and chronic blood loss.
Iron deficiency	Hypochromic-microcytic indices, poikilocytosis, pencil forms, and hyperplastic marrow with increased normoblasts. Absence of stainable iron in the marrow in children older than 2 years.
Vitamin B_{12} and folate deficiency	Large macrocytes, occasional nucleated red blood cells (RBCs), and multisegmented neutrophils. Megaloblastic erythropoiesis in the marrow.
Hemolytic	These types of anemia may be congenital or acquired. They are characterized by a low RBC count, low hemoglobin values, circulating free hemoglobin and possibly hemoglobinuria, elevated reticulocyte count and bilirubin, decreased serum haptoglobin, abnormal peripheral blood smear, and possibly hepatomegaly and splenomegaly. Etiologies include blood group incompatibility (ABO/Rho), hereditary spherocytosis, hereditary nonspherocytic hemolytic anemia, sickle cell anemia, thalassemia, G-6-PD deficiency, pyruvate kinase deficiency, autoim-

Hemolytic (cont'd)	mune hemolytic anemia, drugs, infection, hemolytic-uremic syndrome, and collagen-vascular diseases.
Defective Red Cell Production	This may be caused by infection, drugs, hypo-plastic and aplastic anemias, megaloblastic anemias, hypothyroidism, tumors, leukemia, hepatic disease, bone disease, lipid storage diseases, Letterer-Siwe disease, and uremia.
Infection—Chronic	Normochromic-normocytic; occasionally hypochromic-microcytic. Acute infection may produce a hemolytic anemia. There is thought to be a toxic suppression of the bone marrow as well as decreased RBC survival time with chronic infections.

Cause of Anemia	Pallor	Jaundice	Splenomegaly	Hepatomegaly	Pancytopenia	Normal MCV	Low MCV	Family History of Anemia	Low RB Count	Low Ferritin	Rise in Circulating Free Hgb	Petechiae/Purpura	Abnormal Clotting Factor	Poikilocytes	Schistocytes	Macrocytes	Microcytes	Hyperplastic Marrow	Hypoplastic Marrow	Nucleated RBCs
Acute blood loss	3	0	0	0	0	4	0	0	2	1	0	1-4	0	0	0	0	0	0-4	0	(4)
Chronic blood loss	3	0	0	1	0	1	*	0	*	3	0	1	0	2-4	0	0	*	4	0	1-2
Nutritional (Fe deficiency)	3	0	1	0	0	0	4	0	4	4	0	1	0	3	0	0	4	4	0	0
Vitamin B$_{12}$ and folate deficiency	3	0	0	0	1	0	0	1	4	1	0	0	0	0	0	4	0	4	0	3
Hemolytic	3	3	3	1	1	1	0	3	4	0	4	4	0	2	4	1	0	4	0	4
Defective RBC production	3	0	0	0	2	1	0	3	4	0	0	1	0	0	0	0	0	0	4	0
Acute infection	3	0	*	*	0	1	1	0	1	3	0	1	0	*	0	0	1	4	1	3
Chronic infection	3	0	*	*	0	1	3	0	3	3	0	0	0	0	*	0	3	0	4	0

MCV, mean corpuscular volume.

Ataxia

Ataxia is the loss of the power of muscle coordination. It may be manifested in many ways. A common presentation is an uncoordinated gait, which is usually described as "drunken." The onset may be acute or chronic. The child is unable to maintain balance, appears clumsy, or may not be able to remain upright in a sitting position.

The examiner should search the history for familial etiologies. Questions should also focus on prior infections and the ingestion of drugs or foreign substances. The physical examination should include a complete neurological examination, as well as examination of other systems that may yield evidence of systemic involvement.

Drug Reaction	This may occur with antihistamines, chlordiazepoxide, colistin, diazepam, phenytoin, indomethacin, meprobamate, streptomycin, ethanol, and vincristine.
Hypoglycemia	Other symptoms associated with hypoglycemia are vertigo, pallor, diaphoresis, tachypnea, tachycardia, tremor, convulsions, and coma.
Cerebellitis	This is a postinfectious encephalitis characterized by ataxia, nystagmus, and tremors; it may follow acute viral infections. A common etiology is varicella.
Weakness and Ataxia	Weakness may be mistaken for ataxia—the loss of coordinated movements—since the gait is unstable owing to weak postural muscles.
Acute Cerebellar Ataxia	This is characterized by hypotonia, decreased deep tendon reflexes, nystagmus, intention tremor, and ataxia.

Ataxia–Telan-giectasia	Neurological manifestations begin in infancy. Walking begins late and is always ataxic. Other symptoms are intention tremor, nystagmus, and dysarthria. The eye movements are characteristic (normal involuntary control but loss of voluntary control). After 5 years of age, telangiectasias may be evident on the bulbar conjunctivae and skin.
Friedreich's Ataxia	Skeletal deformities may occur with Friedreich's ataxia. They include pes cavus, hammer toe, and scoliosis. Cardiac disturbances are failure and arrhythmias. Neurological disturbances are ataxia, dysarthria, nystagmus, intention tremor, loss of deep tendon reflexes, and distal weakness. The classic triad is ataxia, a positive Babinski sign, and absent ankle jerks.
Other Causes of Ataxia	Heat stroke, hypothyroidism, abetalipoproteinemia, Hartnup disease, maple syrup urine disease, disseminated sclerosis, mumps, varicella, head injuries, and hysteria.

Cause of Ataxia	Nystagmus	Weakness	Head Tremor	Tremor	Decreased Muscle Tone	Delayed Development	Dysarthria	Skeletal Deformity	Skin Manifestations	Decreased Deep Tendon Reflex	Upgoing Positive Babinski Sign	Family History	Diaphoresis
Drugs	3–4	2	0	3	2	0	1	0	2	2	1	0	1
Hypoglycemia	1	4	0	3	2	0	0	0	0	1	1	0	4
Cerebellitis	1–3	0	1–3	1–3	0	0	0–2	0	0	0	0	0	0
Weakness	0	4	0	3	0	0	0	0	0	0	0	0	0
Acute cerebellar ataxia	2	1	2	4	4	0	0	0	0	4	0	0	0
Ataxia-telangiectasia	4	0	0	0	2	4	4	0	4	0	0	4	0
Friedreich's ataxia	3	4	0	0	3	0	4	4	0	4	4	4	0
Brain tumor	1	*	0	1–4	1	0	1	0	0	1–4	1–4	0	0
Hysteria	0	3	2	0	0	0	0	0	0	0	0	0	1

Blood Pressure Elevation

Blood pressure elevation occurs with considerable frequency in childhood (1.4% to 11%). Early recognition and treatment of pathological hypertension may avert many of the sequellae. Children 3 years of age and older should have their blood pressure routinely screened on an annual basis. The cuff should cover approximately ⅔ of the child's upper arm and should snugly encircle the arm without overlapping itself. Deflation of the cuff should occur at a rate of approximately 2–3 mm Hg/sec. In smaller infants and neonates, a flush or Doppler technique may be utilized to determine the mean arterial pressure. If an elevation of blood pressure is discovered in a single extremity, it should also be determined in the other arm and the legs (both supine and upright). Blood pressure elevation greater than the 95th percentile for age on three separate occasions is abnormal. The clinical features of elevated blood pressure are nonspecific and diffuse. Cephalgia and epistaxis is unusual in childhood hypertension and their presence usually signifies significant end-organ pathology. Blurred vision, seizures or congestive heart failure are rare and usually associated with secondary forms of hypertension. Their presence should alert the clinician to focus on known potential anatomical changes.

High Normal Blood Pressure	In the asymptomatic child, any casual blood pressure measurement (systolic and/or diastolic) above the 95th percentile for age and sex is considered to be high normal blood pressure. Two subsequent determinations of blood pressure should be performed at 2 to 3 week

High Normal Blood Pressure (cont'd)	intervals (by the same examiner, using the same equipment).
Sustained Elevated Blood Pressure	In the asymptomatic child (and in the absence of end-organ damage), elevation of the blood pressure above the 95th percentile for age and sex on three separate occasions separated by 2 to 3 week intervals is termed sustained elevated blood pressure.
Fixed Elevated Blood Pressure	Fixed elevated blood pressure is present in a child with prior diagnosis of sustained elevated blood pressure who, after follow-up for approximately 1 year, continuously has blood pressure measurements exceeding the 90th percentile (with a majority of the recordings above the 95th percentile). It is also considered in a newly presenting patient who is symptomatic from the elevated blood pressure and usually has pressure readings at least 10 to 20 mm Hg above the 95th percentile for age and sex.
Etiologies of Fixed Elevated Blood Pressure	Primary hypertension and secondary hypertension associated with renal, cardiovascular, endocrine, or collagen-vascular disease, CNS abnormalities, drugs, toxins, burns, orthopedic procedures, genitourinary procedures, hypercalcemia, porphyria, dysautonomia, and Stevens-Johnson syndrome.

Bloody Stools

The appearance of blood in the stool is usually a cause of great alarm. The parents usually seek early medical attention or advice. The problem may be either trivial or severe.

It must be determined at the outset whether the red color that appeared in the stool was, in fact, blood. The stool must be accurately described as to color, consistency, and location of the "blood." Blood coating a normally-formed stool carries a different significance than blood mixed with mucus in a diarrhea stool.

The quantity of the blood must be determined. The parents must be questioned about the presence of painful defecation and constipation. Is there abdominal pain? Is there an associated fever? Has there been vomiting? What is the exact color of the stool? What has recently been ingested? Have there been any recent nosebleeds? Is any other member of the family ill?

On physical examination the anus must be completely inspected, and a rectal examination must be performed. Signs of an acute abdomen must be searched for, as well as any evidence of abdominal trauma. The urine should be evaluated in addition to the stool, since a bloody diaper may result from hematuria, as well as hematochezia.

Swallowed Maternal Blood	Swallowed maternal blood may appear in the stool of a newborn infant. The color is variable; it may be red, or it may be black and slimy, mixed with meconium. The patient looks well. The Apt test is used to differentiate fetal from maternal blood. (The Apt test is described in the chapter on hematemesis.)

Anal Fissures	An anal fissure is the most common cause of bloody stools in infants and children. There may be a history of constipation. The parents may state that defecation appears painful to the child. The blood is usually bright red and small in volume. It may appear to coat the outside of the stool. The fissure may be seen on inspection of the anus. The fissure usually results from the passage of a hard stool, or it may be secondary to accidental trauma (for example, during taking of rectal temperatures). Chronic anal fissures should alert the examiner to the possibility of an underlying organic disease process. Anal fissures may also be a sign of sexual molestation. An anal fissure in the presence of lax sphincter tone (in the absence of organic disease) should prompt the examiner to search for other signs and symptoms of child abuse.
Milk Allergy	The amount of blood seen in the stool with milk allergy is variable. There may be no gross blood present, or the amount may be minimal. The color is usually bright red. There may be a history of intermittent colic, vomiting, diarrhea, angioedema, eczema, asthma, or other allergic manifestations. The history will usually reveal the ingestion of a cow's milk product. The physical examination is usually unremarkable, unless evidence of a recent allergic reaction is present, e.g., asthma or eczema. These infants may become severely anemic; therefore, a blood cell count should be obtained on all infants with suspected milk allergy.
Hemorrhagic Disease of the Newborn	Bloody stools, as well as other manifestations (petechiae, ecchymosis, hematemesis, nasal bleeding, and abnormal coagulation studies), are usually observed.

Necrotizing Enterocolitis (NEC)	Necrotizing enterocolitis (NEC) is primarily a disease of the premature and stressed newborn fed with artificial formula. There is usually a history of hypoxia, idiopathic respiratory distress syndrome (hyaline membrane disease), umbilical artery catheterization, and nasogastric or nasal jejunal tube feedings. Bloody diarrheal stools, hematemesis, abdominal distention, and shock are other manifestations of NEC. These newborns appear extremely ill, and vigorous therapy must be instituted rapidly. The stool usually contains gross blood, mucus, and pus.
Gastritis	Gastric inflammation and irritation from any cause can result in gastrointestinal hemorrhage. The placement of nasogastric tubes can cause inflammation and irritation of the gastric mucosa, resulting in bleeding. Hemoglobin is irritating to the gastrointestinal tract, and mass peristaltic movements may result. In adults, upper gastrointestinal bleeding usually results in melena, and no gross blood is seen in the stool. In children, however, because of the mass peristaltic movements, upper gastrointestinal bleeding can cause bright red blood to appear in the stool.
Gastroenteritis	Any gastrointestinal infection can cause blood to appear in the stool. If the agent invades the mucosa or causes mucosal ulceration or friability, bleeding may occur. Bacterial or parasitic pathogens may be the etiological agents. Viruses play a major role in the etiology of childhood diarrhea. The incidence of hematochezia in cases of viral etiology is considerably less than in those of bacterial or parasitic etiology. Symptoms frequently associated with gastroenteritis are vomiting, loose mucopurulent stools, abdominal pain, decrease in appe-

Gastroenteritis (cont'd)	tite, and fever. The onset is usually acute. Dehydration and weight loss may rapidly ensue. Anemia may occur, especially in the presence of chronic parasitic infection.
Polyps	Intestinal polyps in children are usually idiopathic; however, there is a genetic and familial form of the disease. The polyps may become symptomatic at any age. The amount of blood present in the stool is usually small, although moderate amounts of blood may occur; the blood is bright red in color. There is usually no associated abdominal pain. There may be intermittent mucoid diarrhea. The diagnosis of intestinal polyps is made by barium enema, endoscopy, or upper gastrointestinal X-ray series.
Intussusception	Bloody stools may or may not be present with intussusception. Bloody stools usually occur late in the disease process. When blood is present, the stools are most frequently described as "currant jelly." Children with this condition are usually less than 2 years of age, but intussusception can occur in older children as well. There is an acute onset of colicky abdominal pain. The child may draw the knees up to the chest and scream with pain. These episodes are paroxysmal; between episodes of pain, the child is lethargic. Affected children frequently look very ill. A barium enema is both diagnostic and therapeutic. If the barium enema fails to reduce the intussusception, surgery is indicated.
Meckel's Diverticulum	The amount of blood in the stool is usually large. There is an acute onset of hematochezia. The patient may be pale and in shock, and will look very ill. Abdominal pain is not remarkable, and at times there is no pain. Children

Meckel's Diverticulum (cont'd)	less than 2 years of age are most commonly affected. A radioactive isotope scan may show the Meckel's diverticulum if ectopic gastric mucosa is present; otherwise, diagnosis is usually made by laparotomy.
Ulcerative Colitis and Crohn's Disease	The bleeding may be gross or occult. Diarrhea is usually present. Crohn's disease is additionally characterized by anorexia, weight loss, and abdominal pain. In ulcerative colitis, tenesmus and abdominal pain are present; however, anorexia and weight loss are usually absent.
Other Causes of Bloody Stools	Proctitis, stress ulcer, duplications, hemangiomas, peptic ulcer, Henoch-Schönlein purpura, esophagitis, esophageal varices, hemorrhoids, foreign bodies, and hemolytic-uremic syndrome.

Cause of Bloody Stools	Anorexia	Fever	Abdominal Pain	Mucopurulent Stool	History of Invasive Procedures	Anemia	Shock	Abdominal Distention	Skin Manifestations	Vomiting	Diarrhea	Rectal/Anal Pain	Volume of Blood	Constipation	Apt Test	Patient's Appearance	Stool Color
Swallowed maternal blood	0	0	0	0	0	0	0	0	0	1	1	0	3	0	4	0	4
Anal fissures	0	0	0	0	0	0	0	0	0	0	0	4	4	4	0	0	4
Milk allergy	1	1	1	2*	0	3*	1*	0	2	4	4	4	0	0	0	0	2
Hemorrhagic disease of newborn	1	2	0	0	0	4	2	3	4	1	0	0	0	0	0	4	2
Necrotizing enterocolitis	3	3	3	4	3	3	4	4	0	3	0	0	0	0	0	4	3
Gastritis	0	1	0	0	0	1	0	0	0	4	4	0	0	0	0	0	1
Acute gastroenteritis	2	3	4	1	0	0	1	0	0	3	4	0	0	0	0	2	1
Intestinal polyps	0	0	(4)	0	0	0	0	0	4	0	0	0	0	0	0	0	2
Intussusception	2	1	4	0	0	0	1	2	0	3	0	1	0	3	0	4	4
Meckel's diverticulum	1	1	2	0	0	1–4	0–4	1	0	0	0	0	2–4	0	0	0	2

(continued)

Cause of Bloody Stools (cont'd)	Anorexia	Fever	Abdominal Pain	Mucopurulent Stool	History of Invasive Procedures	Anemia	Shock	Abdominal Distention	Skin Manifestations	Vomiting	Diarrhea	Rectal/Anal Pain	Volume of Blood	Constipation	Apt Test	Patient's Appearance	Stool Color
Inflammatory bowel disease	2	3	4	4	0	3	0	2	0–2	0	4	0	0	0	0	2	2
Peptic ulcer	2	1	4	0	0	3	1	2	0	3	3	0	2	0	0	0	1–4
Henoch-Schönlein purpura	1	1	3	0	0	0	0	0	4	1	1	0	1	1	0	4	1
Foreign body	1	0	2	0	0	0	0	4	0	0	0	4	0	4	0	0	4
Hemolytic uremic syndrome	1	1	2	0	0	4	1	0	4	1	3	0	0	0	0	2	1

Cephalgia

Headache, as an isolated symptom, is not common in infants and children. Furthermore, since headache is a subjective symptom, one cannot prove or disprove its presence. Associated signs and symptomatology may yield evidence of organic pathology; therefore, a thorough history and physical examination may give more information than a multitude of sophisticated laboratory examinations. Questions that should be asked are: When did the headache first begin? What particular sensations does the headache give? What makes it better? What makes it worse? How long does the headache last? Is there associated vomiting, sweating, a visual problem, or dizziness? Is the headache localized or does it radiate? Has there been previous trauma? Has there been a fever? Is the patient taking any drugs? When was the patient's last meal? Does the patient wear glasses? Is there a history of allergy? When was the patient's last menstrual period?

A complete neurological examination is essential. A search should be made for meningeal signs. The eye grounds and visual fields must be checked. A complete ear, nose, and throat examination must be performed. Blood pressure determination is essential and should be done, whether or not the patient is having a headache at the time. The skull should be palpated, and a transillumination of the sinuses and skull should be performed.

Fever	Fever is one of the most common causes of headache during childhood. The fever may come from a multitude of etiologies. Infections of the central nervous system (encephalitis, meningitis, and abscess) may be associated

Fever (cont'd)	with headache as a primary symptom. Headache can occur secondarily when the etiology of fever is outside the central nervous system, e.g., otitis media pharyngitis, pneumonia, tumor, or heat stroke. There may be associated myalgia, cervical adenopathy, or other signs and symptoms of infection.
Psychological	Psychophysiological cephalgia is common, especially in adolescents. Such headaches are relatively uncommon in the 5- to 12-year-olds although they may occur in this age group, they are usually attention-seeking ploys or may result from imitation of an adult. Cephalgia in this age group may be associated with school problems, which should be searched for in the history. Headaches in the adolescent period and psychological headaches in the 5- to 12-year-old age group may be a sign of extreme tension and stress.
Ocular Problems	Problems with accommodation and convergence may cause cephalgia in young children. School problems, such as difficulty in reading, may also be linked to cephalgia. Children with the ocular abnormalities tend to sit in the front of the schoolroom. There may be associated diplopia, amblyopia, or dyslexia. Ocular tumors should be sought. Congenital glaucoma may also cause headache and eye pain. Children with congenital glaucoma may have extremely hyperemic conjunctivae; increased intraocular pressure and photophobia are associated with the headache.
Otitis Media	Middle ear problems, such as serous or suppurative otitis media, can cause cephalgia in children. The mastoid air cells may be involved. When mastoiditis is present there may be tenderness to percussion over the mastoid region.

Otitis Media (cont'd)	Cervical adenitis may be present. In nonsuppurative otitis media, visualization of the tympanic membranes may reveal retraction and air-fluid levels. With suppurative otitis media, the landmarks are obscured and there may be bulging of the drum. The color of the drum is extremely variable, as is the presence of a light reflex, and a red ear with normal landmarks should not be considered a case of otitis media until proved so.
Sinusitis	Sinusitis may be a cause of cephalgia in children; the development of the sinuses continues after birth and is not complete until approximately 7 years of age. In sinusitis there may be mucopurulent rhinorrhea and localized tenderness. Transillumination, as well as X-ray examination of the sinuses, may be of some diagnostic value. Inability to transilluminate a sinus does not mean sinusitis is present; however, it should add to suspicion of this condition. Obscuring of the sinuses on X-ray picture is good evidence that sinusitis is present, but bleeding into the sinus may also obscure visualization on X-ray examination.
Cluster Headaches	Cluster headaches are usually seasonal. They are paroxysmal, occur in crops, and the patient has asymptomatic periods between the headache paroxysms. There may be associated rhinorrhea, unilateral epiphoria, and unilateral flushing of the face.
Migraine	Migraine headaches are usually unilateral, and are paroxysmal and throbbing. They may be preceded by an aura. There may be associated nausea and vomiting, and there is frequently a family history of migraine headache. The pain is ordinarily not relieved with analgesics.

Meningitis/ Encephalitis	Both meningitis and encephalitis may present with a headache as the first symptom. There may be associated fever, meningismus, neck pain, and positive Kernig and Brudzinski signs. Frequently, there is associated vomiting. Occasionally, seizures will be present. Children with meningitic or encephalitic cephalgia usually look ill. There may be a history of a prior illness, such as varicella, mumps, otitis media, pneumonia, or rubeola. An abnormal lumbar puncture showing a pleocytosis, decreased sugar content, and positive gram stain or culture signifies bacterial involvement. A pleocytosis in the presence of a normal sugar and protein, with negative cultures and gram stains, may be indicative of aseptic or tuberculous meningitis.
Intracranial Space-Occupying Lesions	Lesions such as abcess, tumor, and collections of blood can be associated with headache as a first symptom. There may be associated fever, focal neurological signs, and vomiting. There may be a history of trauma. There may be signs of increased intracranial pressure. In infancy, the anterior fontanel may bulge if there is increased intracranial pressure. Older children may have diastasis of the sutures. There may be unilateral weakness. Seizures and change in the sensorium may occur.
Other Causes of Cephalgia	Epileptic equivalents, drug reactions, hypertension, dental caries, hunger, nephritis, plumbism, diabetes, sickle cell anemia, von Recklinghausen's disease, leukemia, Sturge-Weber syndrome, and pheochromocytoma.

Cause of Cephalgia	Fever	Lethargy	Weakness	Adenopathy	Generalized	Localized	Character	Wakes Patient	Present on Waking	Increases During Day	Relieved with Analgesic	Relieved with Sleep	Rhinorrhea	Epiphora	Vomiting	Ocular Abnormality	Family History	Interferes with Play	Associated Symptoms
Fever	4	*	*	*	4	0	0	0	0	1	3	1	*	0	*	0	0	*	4
Psychological/tension	0	1	0	0	2	3	2	0	0	3	3	1	0	0	0	0	1	*	*
Ocular	0	0	0	0	0	3	3	0	0	4	1	4	0	0	0	3	0	0	0
Otitis media	4	0	0	2	1	4	0	1	1	0	1	1	0	0	0	0	0	1	1
Sinusitis	3	0	0	0	0	4	0	0	1	0	1	0	0	0	0	0	0	0	1
Cluster headaches	0	0	0	0	1–3	1–4	4	0	0	4	1	0	4	4	0	3	0	3	0
Migraine	0	1	1	0	1	3	4	0	0*	0*	2	4	4	0	1	3	4	4	1–4
CNS infection	4	3	2	0	3	1	0	0	3	0	1	0	0	0	2	0	0	4	4
Intracranial space-occupying lesion	0	0	0	0	2	2	2	1	4	1	1	0	0	0	3	1	0	2	4

Chest Pain

Chest pain is not an uncommon symptom during childhood and adolescence. It carries a different significance in children than in adults.

It is important to ask the child to point to the location of the pain, since secondhand information from the parent may be misleading. The child may point to his epigastrium and call it his chest.

Significant points in the history should be: Past history: Has there been any prior surgery to the chest? Does the patient have asthma or sickle cell disease? Family history: Is there a family member who also has chest pain? Is there heart disease in the family? Location: Exactly where is the pain located? Can the child point to the area with one finger? Character: Exactly what does the pain feel like? Is it made worse by movement? Is it made worse by deep inspiration? Time: When does it occur? What does it keep the patient from doing? Trauma: Have there been any chest injuries?

Examination of the heart and lungs is essential. Is there any evidence of cardiovascular or pulmonary pathology? Chest wall inspection and palpation may yield clues to a more musculoskeletal etiology. Signs of abuse must be looked for by the examiner. Examination of the abdomen may show that the pain is referred to the chest from intraabdominal pathology.

Psychological/ Psychophysiological	The family history may be positive for angina, and the child may imitate the pain as an attention-getting mechanism. The symptoms usually do not fit into any specific pattern. The pain may be recurrent or paroxysmal; it may

Psychological/ Psychophys- iological (cont'd)	be relieved by distraction. Sleep is not dis- turbed. Play periods are not interrupted.
Musculoskele- tal Pain	Musculoskeletal pain is probably the most common cause of chest pain in childhood. The onset is usually sudden. Other illness is absent. Point pain is most frequent. The pain is exacer- bated by movement or inspiratory efforts. Ten- derness may be present. Occasionally, costochondral pain may occur secondary to costochondritis. With the above symptoms, there may be swelling, redness, and heat at the costochondral junction near the sternum.
Bornholm disease (pleu- rodynia)	Bornholm disease is caused by a Coxsackie virus (group B). There are fever, cephalgia, and severe stabbing chest or abdominal pain. Re- spiratory excursions exacerbate the pain. The muscles are frequently swollen and tender. Other members of the family may be affected. There will be recurrences after 2 to 3 days of symptomless periods in 25% of patients.
Trauma	Contusions and rib fractures may cause local- ized chest pain.
Pulmonary Problems *Pneumonia (including pleuritis)*	Isolated pneumonia is not a common cause of chest pain in childhood. If the pleura is in- volved, directly or indirectly, pain will occur. Physical signs of pneumonia may be present. The pain may be exacerbated by deep inspira- tion or cough. There may be asymmetric ex- cursions secondary to splinting. Radiation of pain to the shoulder is not uncommon. Pain referred to the right lower quadrant of the abdomen is frequent with right lower lobe pneumonia.

Pulmonary embolism/ infarction	Pulmonary embolism or infarction is rare in children. The onset is sudden. Frequently, there are dyspnea, tachycardia, tachypnea, and shock. The pain may be substernal or pleuritic and radiate to a shoulder. Frequently, there are no findings on physical examination, but if the embolism or infarction is large enough, breath sounds may be absent, rales may be present, and a pleural friction rub may be heard. The sputum is frequently bloody.
Cardiac Problems *Pericarditis*	The location, intensity, and character of pain in pericarditis are extremely variable. In general, it is dull and poorly localized. It may be referred to the neck or shoulders. The pain may be increased by respiratory excursion or swallowing. Pulsus paradoxus (lowering of the pulse pressure during inspiration) may be present. Heart sounds may be distant. A friction rub may be ausculated anywhere over the precordium. There may be a finding of Ewart sign, consisting of dullness and bronchial breath sounds over the left lower lobe, secondary to obstruction of the left mainstem bronchus by pericardial fluid, resulting in collapse of the left lung.
Esophagus *Esophagitis*	Chest pain secondary to esophageal inflammation is usually substernal and exacerbated by swallowing. There may be associated vomiting or hematemesis. Dysphagia may be present.
Other Causes of Chest Pain	Aspirated foreign bodies, hepatitis, diaphragmatic pain, peritonitis, hemoperitoneum, gall bladder disease, pneumothorax, pulmonary abcess, sickle cell anemia, stretching of the renal capsule, rheumatic disease of the aortic valve, myocardial infarction, hypertrophic

Other Causes of Chest Pain (cont'd)	cardiomyopathy, cystic fibrosis, spleen rupture, left shoulder pain and rupture of the capsule of liver, and right shoulder pain.

Cause of Chest Pain	Disturbs Sleep	Disturbs Play	Onset Acute	Increases with Movement	Increases with Inspiration	Cough	Local Swelling	Tenderness	Fever	Associated Symptoms	Radiation	Tachypnea	Friction Rub	Increases with Swallowing	Dysphagia
Psychophysiological	0–2	0	4	0	1–4	1–4	0	0	0	1–4	0	0	0	0	0
Musculoskeletal (pleurodynia)	3	3	4	4	4	0	2	4	1–4	0	0	0	0	0	0
Musculoskeletal (trauma)	3	4	4	3	3	1	4	4	0	1	1	2	0	0	0
Pneumonia	2	3	2–3	0	3	3	0	0	2–4	1–3	2	4	1	0	0
Embolism	3	3	4	1	3	3	0	0	1	1	1	3	2	0	0
Pericarditis	3	3	3	0	1	0	0	0	1	3	3	2	4	0	0
Esophagitis	1	1	0	0	0	1	0	0	1	2	2	0	0	4	4
Foreign body aspiration	3	3	4	0	4	3	0	0	1	1	0	3	0	0	0
Pneumothorax	3	3	4	0	4	3	0	0	1	3	0	3	1	0	0
Sickle cell anemia	3	3	3	3	3	3	3	3	3	4	2	3	2	0	0

Child Abuse and Neglect

A 2-year-old boy is brought to the emergency room of a local hospital. The patient's mother states that the child injured himself in a fall from a couch. Physical and X-ray examinations reveal a spiral fracture of the left humerus, healing fractures of the right radius and ulna, and a recent fracture of the right parietal bone.

Such a case illustrates one of the most important decision points in the evaluation of an abused or neglected child. Is there a discrepancy between the history and the injuries? Can the extent of the injuries be explained by the presenting history? Are there bizarre or conflicting explanations of the injuries? If so, child abuse should be suspected.

There are many forms of child abuse and neglect. Physical abuse is the most obvious form and usually the easiest to diagnose. Psychological abuse, sexual abuse, malnutrition (nonorganic failure to thrive), and emotional deprivation are more subtle and more difficult to diagnose. It must be stressed that it is not the health care provider's responsibility to prove or disprove abuse or neglect. The provider's responsibility lies in reporting suspicions to the appropriate city, county, or state agency and, of utmost importance, in the protection of the child from further injury.

Physical Child Abuse	Physical child abuse should be suspected if the patient presents with multiple cuts, bruises, and abrasions (especially in unusual locations and in various stages of healing), cigarette burns, human bites, strap marks, cord marks, multiple hematomas, multiple fractures in various stages of healing, spiral fractures, unexplained subdural hematoma, bizarre or

Physical Child Abuse (cont'd)	conflicting explanations of physical injuries, injuries inconsistent with the history given, and any *pattern* of recurring minor injuries.
Sexual Abuse	Sexual molestation of children does not only involve direct sexual contact between genitalia or penetration. It includes any utilization of children for the sexual gratification of an adult. This might take the form of fondling genitalia, oral/genital contact, forcing a child to view a sexually explicit act, sexual exploitation, and child pornography. It may be difficult to diagnose, since the vast majority of cases present to the health care practitioner without physical evidence of abuse. Several newer methods of diagnosis are being tested, including distance of labial separation in females (to diagnose penetration of the vagina). Lax anal sphincter tone may indicate anal penetration. Any sexually transmitted disease cultured from the oropharynx, vagina, urethra, or rectum in a prepubertal child is prima-facie evidence of child sexual molestation. Sexually explicit coloring books and anatomically correct dolls are being used to assist in the diagnosis. It is important to remember that children rarely lie about sexual contact with an adult. If the child admits to being sexually abused or describes the act of molestation, the child must be believed (until it it proved otherwise by appropriate medical evaluation and social service agency investigation).
Child Neglect	Child neglect occurs when the perpetrator of the neglect blatantly disregards the proper or necessary support, education, medical, or other remedial care necessary for a child's well-being. Blatant disregard refers to incidents where the risk of harm to the child is so

Child Neglect (cont'd)	imminent and apparent that it is unlikely a parent or caretaker would expose the child to such obvious danger without exercising precautionary measures to protect the child from harm. Nonorganic failure to thrive is a form of child neglect in which adequate nutrition for normal growth and development is not provided for the child. The child's weight is usually disproportionately low compared to its length and head circumference. The growth velocity is usually low. A period of hospitalization (where the child is fed a normal diet) results in catch-up growth.
Some Diseases Presenting with Symptoms and Signs Resembling Those of Child Abuse or Neglect	Syphilis, scurvy, infantile cortical hyperostosis, osteogenesis imperfecta, coagulopathies/blood dyscrasias, meningococcemia, and mongolian spots.

Coma

Coma is a state of unconsciousness with many varied etiologies. The history is almost always secondhand. Pertinent information must be obtained rapidly. Ingestion: Has the patient been on any medication or taken any drugs? Trauma: Have there been any recent injuries or accidents? Prior illnesses: Is there a history of diabetes? Does the patient have a seizure disorder? Was the patient ill prior to the unconsciousness?

Physical examination should focus on evidence of trauma, signs of shock, focal neurological signs, and evidence of drug, alcohol, or poison ingestion.

Hypoglycemia	Hypoglycemia from any cause can result in coma. The history may be revealing, as in the case of a diabetes mellitus patient taking insulin. Other symptoms of hypoglycemia include tachycardia, palpitations, tachypnea, diaphoresis, weakness, disorientation, tremor, and convulsions.
Ketotic Hypoglycemia	Ketotic hypoglycemia occurs in children 18 months to 10 years of age; the onset is usually before 5 years of age. Children with this type of hypoglycemia are frequently small for their gestational age. The attacks are paroxysmal and tend to occur in the morning, after a fast or during illness. A symptomatic attack may be precipitated by feeding the child a ketogenic diet.
Diabetic Ketoacidosis	The history may or may not be positive for diabetes. Coma is a frequent symptom, with other frequent symptoms including weakness,

Diabetic Ketoacidosis (cont'd)	nausea, vomiting, dehydration, polyuria, confusion, tachypnea (later, Kussmal respirations), and convulsions.
Seizure Disorder	Coma may characterize postictal states. Major motor seizures need not precede the period of coma. There may be an associated Todd paralysis.
Drugs/Poisons	Drugs and poisons, taken either accidentally or intentionally, can be etiologic for coma. Barbiturates, tranquilizers, morphine derivatives, and similar agents are frequently involved. Alcohol must always be considered. Drugs may also cause hypoglycemia. This is true for maternal sulfonylurias taken during the last trimester of pregnancy, and for alcohol, salicylates, and propranolol. Jamaican vomiting sickness, secondary to drinking "bush tea" (tea made from the unripe fruit of the achee) can cause vomiting, prostration, lethargy, hypoglycemia, convulsion, and coma.
Head Injuries	The history is usually positive for trauma. Concussions are characterized by a period of unconsciousness or amnesia following trauma to the head. Intracranial bleeding, such as subdural hematoma, may cause coma. Progressive focal neurological signs are usually present.
Central Nervous System Infection	Meningitis and encephalitis, regardless of the etiology, may cause alternating states of consciousness, confusion, fever, meningismus, convulsion, or focal neurological signs and symptoms.
Other Causes of Coma	Sepsis, hypovolemia, anaphylaxis, uremia, hypernatremia, increased intracranial pressure, hysteria, hepatitis, and Reye's syndrome.

Cause of Coma

	Head Trauma	Abnormal Laboratory Test Results	Abnormal CSF	Hypoglycemia	Seizures	Vomiting	Hypertension	Prior Infection
Trauma	4	2	1	0	2	2	0	0
CNS infection	1	4	4	0	2	2	0	2
Renal disorder	0	4	0	1	1	3	3	0
Diabetic ketoacidosis	0	4	1	0	1	3	0	2
Reye's syndrome	0	4	4	3	2	4	0	3
Medication ingestion	0	3	0	1	2	2	0	0

Constipation/Infrequent Stools

Constipation is a common problem bringing children to a pediatrician. When present for a long period of time, it is very difficult to resolve.

To most persons, constipation means infrequency of defecation. Constipation, however, refers to hard dry stools that mainly contain solids and hold very little water, as well as infrequency. The condition is commonly, but not necessarily, associated with infrequent defecation.

Specific questions to be asked are: What is the child's normal frequency of bowel movements? Has there been a change in the consistency of the stool? Does defecation appear to be painful? Is there blood in the stool? What are the feeding habits? Exactly what is included in the diet? Is the child toilet trained? What is the color of the stool? Is there any fecal incontinence?

Examination of the rectum, anus, and abdomen is most important.

Newborn	
Intestinal obstruction by meconium (meconium ileus)	Most commonly seen in cystic fibrosis; however, 10% of patients do not have cystic fibrosis. Symptoms begin between 24 and 48 hours of life. Abdominal distention, poor eating, and bilious vomiting may occur. Symptoms may appear before 24 hours if a complication (such as perforation) is present. A mass may be palpated. Plain abdominal radiographs may show uneven, dilated loops of bowel, few air-fluid levels, and a bubbly, granular density. Microcolon from disuse may be seen on barium enema.
Small left colon syndrome	Disturbance of peristalsis. Seen more commonly in infants of diabetic mothers. The in-

Small left co-lon syndrome (cont'd)	fants may pass a sticky plug of mucus followed by flatus and liquid meconium.
Atresia/ stenosis	Signs and symptoms of intestinal obstruction include maternal hydramnios, bilious vomiting, and abdominal distention. Failure to pass meconium is more common with low obstruction. With a high obstruction, e.g., duodenal atresia, meconium may be passed. Atresia/ stenosis is more common in the premature infant, and in cases where other congenital anomalies are present.
Imperforate anus	No anal opening is seen on physical examination. An anal dimple is usually present. A fistulous opening may be seen in the perineum; however, the opening may be vulvar in the female or urethral in the male. A cutaneous collection of meconium in the perineal area is an important physical finding.
Functional ileus of the newborn	More common in the premature infant. Sepsis, pneumonia, electrolyte imbalance, and metabolic abnormalities can cause functional ileus. Signs and symptoms of intestinal obstruction may be present in the absence of anatomical obstruction.
Hirsch-sprung's disease	The majority of cases will present within the first seven days of life. There will be a failure to pass meconium, abdominal distention, bilious vomiting, and poor feeding. If not diagnosed in the first weeks of life, the disease may eventually produce severe diarrhea, with failure to thrive, vomiting, and abdominal distention. Fifty percent of infants with Hirschsprung's disease develop enterocolitis, and diarrhea usually indicates the presence of concomitant enterocolitis. Older children with Hirschsprung's disease manifest failure to

Hirsch- sprung's disease (cont'd)	thrive, severe constipation, foul, ribbon-like stools, enlarged abdomen with venous patterns, and visible peristalic waves. Fecal masses may be palpated. Hypoproteinemia, anemia, and failure to thrive are also present. The anus and rectum are devoid of fecal material on digital rectal examination. The canal may feel narrow and tight. Plain X-ray films may show gaseous distention. Barium enema may show a narrowed distal segment and a dilated proximal segment of colon. Residual barium, present 12 to 48 hours after the initial examination, suggests megacolon. Rectal biopsy is the best method of diagnosis. The demonstration of aganglionosis confirms the diagnosis.
Meconium plug syn- drome	The patient may exhibit signs and symptoms of intestinal obstruction. Infants with this condition may pass a sticky white plug of mucus followed by flatus and liquid meconium. The presentation may be similar to the small left colon syndrome.
Infancy and Childhood *Common eti- ologies for constipation and infre- quent stools*	Complete breast feeding, undiluted cow's milk, insufficient fluid or sugar in the diet, mismanagement of toilet training, laxative abuse, and anal fissures (painful defecation and bloody stools).
Less Common Etiologies *Congenital hypothy- roidism*	Umbilical hernia, persistent jaundice, constipation, low T_4 and high thyroid stimulating hormone (TSH) levels may be present.
Lead poisoning	Associated findings may be a history of pica, elevated blood lead and erythrocyte protoporphyrin levels, scattered lead opacities on flat

Lead poisoning (cont'd)	plate of the abdomen, lead lines on X-ray film of the long bones, basophilic stippling of red cells, seizures, developmental disabilities, learning disorders, and neuropathies.
Infantile botulism	Infantile botulism occurs after the ingestion of clostridial spores. This differs from the other form of botulism, in that the toxin is not pre-formed and the infant ingests the organism directly. Constipation is the most striking and consistent first symptom of infantile botulism. Hypotonia and weakness may follow. The cry is weak. With supportive therapy, children with this condition have a good prognosis. Management of fluid and electrolyte problems, as well as respiratory support, is essential.
Other Etiologies for Constipation and Infrequent Stools	Metabolic conditions associated with polyuria, diabetes insipidus, renal tubular acidosis, hypercalcemia, and hyperkalemia.

Cause of Constipation/Infrequent Stools	Stool Consistency	Decreased Frequency	Pain (Anal/Rectal)	Bloody Stool	Toilet Trained	Stool Color	Previously Normal Stool	Associated Symptoms	Abdominal Distention
Meconium ileus	(4)	4	0	0	0	0	0	4	4
Meconium plug	4	3	3	0	0	4	0	3	2
Small left colon	4	4	0	0	0	1	0	2	2
Atresia/stenosis	0	4	0	0	0	1	0	4	2
Imperforate anus	(4)	4	0	0	0	4	3	4	3
Functional ileus of newborn	0	4	1	1	0	0	2	4	3
Hirschsprung's disease	2	3	0	0	4	0	0	3	2
Fluid deficit	3	2	0	0	0–4	0	2–4	1	0
Dietary	2	3	0	0	3	0	3	2	0
Toileting problems	4	4	4	3	0–4	2	4	*	0
Anal fissures	1–4	4	4	4	2	1	3	0	0
Hypothyroidism	4	4	0	0	0	0	0	4	0
Lead poisoning	0	3	0	0	3	0	3	4	0

Cough

Coughing is a normal reflex that functions to clear the tracheobronchial tree. The stimulus may be exogenous (e.g., foreign bodies, dust, smoke) or endogenous (e.g., increased mucus production, airway edema, irritation from pneumonia, bronchitis). Coughing may be acute or chronic; paroxysmal coughing may disturb eating or sleep habits.

The following features are important in obtaining the history: Time of onset: Exactly when did the coughing begin? Fever: Was the patient ill prior to the onset of the cough? Upper airway problems: Is there any nasal congestion? Are there known allergies? Relationship to food? Was the patient eating at the time of onset? Mucus production: Is the cough productive? Tuberculosis: Is there a family history of tuberculosis? Has the patient had a positive skin test for tuberculosis? Congenital heart disease: Is there known cardiovascular disease? Asthma: Is there a history of asthma or paroxysmal wheezing?

Examination of the lungs should focus on the presence or absence of rales, ronchi, upper airway sounds, wheezing, equality and character of breath sounds, and percussion dullness. The heart should be examined for the presence of murmurs and extra sounds. The liver and spleen should be checked for palpability. Is there generalized or localized lymphadenopathy? Is there nasal congestion or rhinorrhea? Is the throat red? Is there a skin rash? Is there otitis media? Is there conjunctivitis?

Upper Respiratory Tract Infection	Cough frequently occurs during simple upper respiratory tract infection. Rhinorrhea, fever, sore throat, or ear pain may be associated. The lungs are clear; however, there may be

Upper Respiratory Tract Infection (cont'd)	transmitted upper airway sounds. The etiology is usually viral, and the course is self-limited.
Lower Respiratory Tract Infection *Viral pneumonia*	Children with viral pneumonia may present with varied degrees of symptoms. Rales may be diffuse or localized. If atelectasis occurs, breath sounds will decrease. The patient may be tachypneic and febrile, and may manifest varying degrees of respiratory distress.
Bacterial pneumonia	In general, bacterial pneumonia presents with more significant and severe symptoms than viral pneumonia. The onset may be abrupt or insidious; fever and prostration usually occur. Lobar consolidation with decreased breath sounds and dullness to percussion may be found. There may be a lag in the respiratory excursion on the affected side.
Bronchiolitis	Bronchiolitis is usually preceded by symptoms of a simple upper respiratory tract infection. Fever is low grade. A cough gradually develops, along with respiratory distress. Wheezing is characteristic. Rales may be heard at the end of inspiration and during early expiration. Breath sounds may be decreased.
Pertussis	Pertussis has three stages and may last from 6 to 8 weeks. The symptoms of the first stage are those of an upper respiratory tract infection (cough, runny nose, and fever). This progresses to severe paroxysmal coughing, with associated facial redness, cyanosis, bulging eyes, and an expression of anxiety. The coughing paroxysm is followed by a characteristic inspiratory whoop. Facial petechiae, vomiting, and exhaustion may occur. The convalescent period is characterized by a slow resolution of the paroxysms. Characteristic symptoms may not

Pertussis (cont'd)	occur in children previously immunized or infants less than 6 months old.
Laryngo-tracheo-bronchitis (LTB)	Symptoms of an upper respiratory tract infection occur during the first few days. These progress to a brassy cough, respiratory distress, and varying degrees of inspiratory stridor. There may be rales, ronchi, and a decrease in breath sounds. Onset of viral croup is relatively insidious, as opposed to epiglottis, where onset is abrupt.
Foreign Body	The history may be positive for ingestion of peanuts, popcorn, hot dogs or a foreign body. The cough is acute in onset, and patients are well prior to cough onset. Breath sounds are usually diminished in the lobe where the foreign body is lodged. There may be asymmetrical expansion of the chest during respiratory excursions. Chest pain may be present. Fluoroscopy, as well as inspiratory/expiratory chest X-ray films, may be diagnostic. On inspiration the chest X-ray film may appear normal. On expiration there may be overexpansion of the involved lung with mediastinal shift away from the side in which the foreign body is lodged. A missed foreign body may present with chronic recurrent coughing, recurrent wheezing, or persistent infiltrates on X-ray examination.
Asthma	Coughing associated with pruritis of the chin, neck, and chest may be the first symptom of an asthmatic paroxysm. Expiratory wheezing, a prolonged expiratory phase of respiration, and rales are characteristic. The attacks are paroxysmal and reversible. There may be varying degrees of respiratory distress.

Rubeola	The characteristic triad of the prodrome of rubeola is cough, coryza, and conjunctivitis. The cough is characteristically barking and brassy, and is invariably present. The prodomal symptoms are followed by fleeting Koplik spots and a morbilliform rash. The degree of symptomatology depends upon the age and immunization status of the patient.
Other Causes of Cough	Parasitic infections, pneumothorax, aspiration pneumonia, smoking, cystic fibrosis, tracheoesophageal fistula, chalasia, hiatal hernia, alpha-1-antitrypsin deficiency, bronchopulmonary dysplasia, and congenital heart disease.

Cause of Cough	Fever	Rhinorrhea	Breath Sounds	Rales	Ronchi	Wheezing	Respiratory Distress	Acute Onset	Paroxysms	Whoop	Facial Petechiae	Stridor	Asymmetrical Chest Expansion	Chest Pain	Abnormal Chest X-ray	Associated Symptoms	Family History
URI	3	4	0	0	0–2	0	0	0	0	0	0	0	0	0	0	4	0
Viral pneumonia	1	3	1	2	0–2	1	3	0	0	0	0	0	1	1	4	3	0
Bacterial pneumonia	4	2	4	4	0–3	1	3	1	0	0	0	0	3	3	4	2	0
Bronchiolitis	1	3	1	3	0	4	3	2	0	0	0	0	0	0	4	3	2
LTB	1	3	2	0	0	2	2	1	0	0	1	4	0	0	2	3	0
Foreign body	0	0	3	1	0	3	4	4	4	0	1	4	4	1	4	1	0
Asthma	0–1	1	4	3	1–3	4	4	3	4	2	0	0	1	1	3	3	4
Rubeola	4	4	0	0	0	0	1	0	0	0	0	0	0	0	2	4	3
Congestive heart failure	0–1	0	4	4	0	0–4	4	1	4	0	0	0	0	0	4	4	0
Pertussis	1	3	0	0	0	0	2	0	4	4	4	0	0	2	0	3	3

Diarrhea

Diarrhea is a frequent complaint in children and has many varied etiologies. The description of the stool is important in formulating a differential diagnosis; new parents may mistakenly interpret a normal stool as a diarrhea stool. The normal formula stool is yellow, seedy, soft, and frequently described as mushy. A normal breast milk stool is slightly looser than a formula stool, and its color is from golden to green.

The frequency of stool will yield information as to the severity of the illness. Six or less stools per day are usual, but a newborn may stool with each feeding because of an active gastrocolic reflex. Infants having loose, watery stools from 6 to 10 times per day are usually not in danger of dehydration, as long as fluid intake is adequate; however, infants that have more than 10 watery stools per day may be in danger of dehydration even if intake is adequate.

Other questions that should be asked are: How long has the child had diarrhea? Is there blood in the stool? What is the relationship of the stool to feedings? Is there associated vomiting? What is the patient's diet? Are any other family members ill? Has the child ingested any foreign substances? Is there fever? Is there abdominal pain? Is the baby thriving?

Because of the numerous etiologies of diarrhea, only the most important will be discussed.

Osmotic Diarrhea	Osmotic diarrhea occurs when there is too large a quantity of sugar in the feeding. The osmotic load to the intestine is then great, and this pulls water into the lumen of the bowel. Children with this type of diarrhea are well and are not malnourished or dehydrated unless the

Osmotic Diarrhea (cont'd)	condition is protracted. These children also eat well, and the physical examination usually shows no abnormalities.
Acute Gastro-enteritis (AGE)	Acute gastroenteritis (AGE) is marked by the acute onset of loose, watery-to-mucoid stools. There may be associated fever, abdominal pain (sometimes colicky), vomiting, and decrease in appetite. Other family members may also be ill. The etiology may be bacterial, viral, parasitic, irritative, or toxic. Blood may appear in the stool if there is mucosal invasion. The abdominal pain and diarrhea are usually increased or prolonged with solid foods. If the patient's intake is poor or vomiting is significant, dehydration may occur. *Dehydration can occur rapidly in children.*
	Food intolerance can also cause AGE. This may be seen in infants after addition of a new food. Older children and adolescents may experience similar symptoms after eating spicy or greasy foods.
	Etiologies of acute gastroenteritis may be viral (e.g., enterovirus or rotavirus infection), bacterial (e.g., *Shigella, Salmonella,* or *E. coli* infection), or parasitic. *Campylobacter jejuni* is almost as common as *Salmonella* in the bacterial etiology of gastroenteritis. The disease is usually self-limiting and mild to moderate in severity. Dehydration usually does not occur. Symptoms usually last 1 week, but abdominal pain may persist for up to 6 weeks. Infection with *Yersinia enterocolitica* occurs during the first 3 years of life. The infection presents as acute gastroenteritis and is difficult to differentiate from other etiologies. In older children, abdominal pain may be the most striking symptom, and the diagnosis may be confused

Acute Gastro-enteritis (AGE) (cont'd)	with acute appendicitis or inflammatory bowel disease.
Food Contami-nation *Staphylo-coccal gas-troenter-itis (food poisoning)*	In staphylococcal gastroenteritis there may be a history of ingestion of a food substance that has been improperly refrigerated during storage. The onset of symptoms occurs between 4 and 6 hours after ingestion of contaminated food. There are nausea, vomiting, abdominal pain, and diarrhea. Frequently, there is a history of other family members also affected.
Botulism	Botulism occurs after the ingestion of a pre-formed toxin of the organism *Clostridium botulinum.* There is usually a history of ingestion of a food substance that has been stored in a vacuum-packed can. The food that was ingested is frequently not cooked, since heating the toxin renders it inactive. The onset of symptoms is usually within 12 to 72 hours after ingestion. There are nausea, vomiting, and diarrhea, followed rapidly by xerostomia, diplopia, blurred vision, and difficulty in swallowing. Dizziness may also occur. There may be increasing muscular weakness that may gradually lead to paralysis of the respiratory musculature. As with other types of "food poisoning," there may be history of other family members involved.
Other Causes of Acute Diarrhea	Antibiotics, allergy, constipation with enco-presis, appendicitis, Hirschsprung's disease, inflammatory bowel disease (ulcerative colitis and Crohn's disease), pseudomembranous enterocolitis, parenteral infection, urinary tract infection, and adrenal insufficiency.
Poor Diet	With an inadequate diet, diarrhea is usually recurrent. Growth and development may be slow. Failure to thrive may be striking. There

Poor Diet (cont'd)	may be a history of frequent dietary changes, and multiple formulas may have been used. The dietary history is important. Children with diarrhea from poor diet will frequently improve and gain weight after being put on an adequate diet in the hospital. Physical examination is frequently unremarkable, except that growth and development may be below the third percentile.
Carbohydrate Intolerance	Carbohydrate intolerance may be primary or secondary. An example of primary carbohydrate intolerance is seen with congenital lactase deficiency. Diarrhea may be severe. Failure to thrive may also be present. These patients usually eat well, but are commonly irritable and frequently colicky. There is no associated vomiting. The patients thrive, and diarrhea resolves, when lactose is removed from the diet. Secondary lactase deficiency is frequently seen in children after an episode of infectious diarrhea; the infection resolves, but the diarrhea continues, and may persist for up to three weeks. Improvement occurs when these children are taken off lactose-containing formulas. The lactase deficiency is temporary, and prolonged use of nonlactose-containing formulas is not necessary.
Milk Allergy	Certain children have a specific allergy to cow's milk protein. These children are irritable, colicky, and have frequent, recurrent loose stools. The stools may be bloody; the child may be anemic; and there may be generalized edema, failure to thrive, and dehydration. The diarrhea resolves with the elim-

Milk Allergy (cont'd)	ination of cow's milk protein from the diet. The child thrives on soy protein formulas.
Parasitic Infections	Unrecognized parasitic infections can be an etiology of chronic diarrhea. The stools may be bloody. There may be abdominal pain. Anemia may be present and there may be failure to thrive.
Other Causes of Chronic Diarrhea	Intestinal polyps, abetalipoproteinemia, acrodermatitis enteropathica, blind loop syndrome, carcinoid tumors, sprue, chronic pancreatitis, cystic fibrosis, enterokinase deficiency, exocrine pancreatic hypoplasia, familial chloride diarrhea, ganglioneuroma, hyperthyroidism, immune deficiency, inflammatory bowel disease, intestinal lymphangiectasis, maternal deprivation syndrome, non-beta-cell pancreatic tumors, marasmus, kwashiorkor, short bowel syndrome, upper small bowel infection or infestation, and Whipple's disease.

Cause of Diarrhea	Stool Character	Frequency	Vomiting	Fever	Family History	Abdominal Pain	Physical Abnormalities	Acute Onset	Chronic	Weakness	Constipation	Abnormal Growth Development	Positive Diet History	FTT	Anemia	Generalized Edema	Joint Pain	Pulmonary Disease
Gastroenteritis (viral)	0	4	3	2	2	1	2	3	0	2	0	0	0	0	0	0	1	0
Gastroenteritis (toxic)	3	3	0	1	0	3	3	4	0	3	0	0	4	0	0	0	0	0
Gastroenteritis (parasitic)	3	2	1	2	2	2	1	2	2	2	1	2	0	1	2	0	0	0
Gastroenteritis (bacterial)	3	3	2	4	2	3	3	3	1	1	0	0	0	0	0	0	0	0
Inadequate diet	0	3	0	0	0	0	2	0	4	2–4	3	2–4	4	4	3	2	0	0
Carbohydrate intolerance	3	3	0	0	4	4	1	4	1–4	1	0	0	4	2	0	0	0	0
Celiac disease	3	3	3	0	3	2	4	1	1–4	4	0	4	4	4	0	3	0	0
Ulcerative colitis	4	3	1	2	3	4	4	2	4	3	0	3	3	3	3	2	0	1
Crohn's disease	3	3	1	3	3	4	4	1	4	3	0	3	3	3	3	0	2	1
Cystic fibrosis	3	3	0	2	1	1	3	1	4	2	0	3	2	3	1	2	2	4
Milk allergy	4	3	3	1	1	3	1	4	1–4	1	0	1	4	2	1	0	0	1

Dyspnea

Dyspnea refers to difficulty in breathing from any cause. The child may complain of trouble breathing, or the parent may state that the child is short of breath. Rapid shallow respirations, "funny" or "noisy" breathing are the usual subjective complaints.

The patient's history should be investigated for prior illnesses and allergy, asthma, heart disease, trauma, and drugs. Could the patient have aspirated a foreign body? Has there been any recent trauma?

Physical examination should focus on the pulmonary, cardiovascular, and nervous systems. A psychosocial evaluation is also important in determining the etiology.

Psychological	Hyperventilation syndrome is characterized by dyspnea, tachypnea, and hyperpnea, resulting in acute respiratory alkalosis. Syncope, tetanic muscle spasms, and paresthesia are common.
Common Causes of Dyspnea	Upper respiratory tract infection, pneumonia, asthma, bronchiolitis, foreign body, acidosis, heart disease, anemia, and drugs—particularly salicylates.
Less Common Causes of Dyspnea	Pleural effusion, emphysema, bronchopulmonary dysplasia, hyaline membrane disease (prematurity), transient tachypnea of the newborn, cysts, pneumothorax, atelectasis, pulmonary agenesis, pulmonary fibrosis, cor pulmonale, diaphragmatic hernia, mediastinal or pulmonary mass, alpha$_1$-antitrypsin deficiency, choanal atresia, chest deformity, trauma, shock, renal failure, and cystic fibrosis.

Dysuria

Dysuria means painful urination. The etiologies are usually confined to the genitourinary tract. It must be remembered that the urinary tract may become involved in certain systemic illnesses; therefore, dysuria may occur as a secondary manifestation.

Historical information is of value in localizing the lesion. Other urinary tract symptoms may be present, including frequency, urgency, incontinence, polyuria, and hematuria. The patient's description of his or her urinary stream is important. Is the stream forceful, or very weak and dribbling? Is there a single stream, or is the stream split?

In infants, there may be crying on passing urine, the diaper may be stained with bloody urine, and urine may be voluntarily held, since the urination is painful. Inspection of the perineum may yield clues to the etiology. Local lesions or irritation external to the urinary tract, such as perineal irritation from a diaper rash, may be the source of the pain.

Urinary Tract Infection	Children may describe dysuria as burning, painful, or hot urine. Fever may be present. Frequency, hesitancy, urgency, incontinence, dribbling, hematuria, and pyuria are other common symptoms.
Urethral Inflammation	Any cause of urethral inflammation can cause dysuria. Hesitancy may be present, but other urinary tract symptoms are usually absent. Some common causes of urethral inflammation are nonspecific or gonococcal urethritis, Reiter's syndrome, diaper rash, local trauma (including child abuse), urethral carbuncle, and balantitis.

Nephritis	Symptoms of urinary tract infection may be present. Hematuria (gross and microscopic) is more commonly associated with nephritis than with urinary tract infection. Nephrotic syndrome and hypertension may occur. Red blood cell casts in the urine are characteristic.
Urethral Stones	Hematuria is very common. Hypertension usually does not occur. Renal colic may be the most striking symptom.
Other Causes of Dysuria	Congenital anomalies of the genital urinary system (e.g., meatal stenosis, urethral valves).

Cause of Dysuria	Fever	Frequency	Hesitancy	Urgency	Gross Hematuria	Microscopic Hematuria	Pyuria	RBC Casts	Abdominal Pain	Flank Pain	Hypertension	Nephrotic Syndrome
Cystitis	2	3	2	3	1-2	3	4	0	4	0	0	0
Urethritis	0	1	4	0	0	0	1	0	0	0	0	0
Pyelonephritis	3	2	0	0	2	3	4	0	1	4	0	0
Glomerulonephritis	1	0	0	0	3	4	2	4	1	1	3	1
Stones (urethral)	1	0	0	0	1	3	2	0	0	4	0	0
Congenital anomalies	0	2	2	2	0	1	1	0	1	0	0	0

Edema

When discussing the differential diagnosis, the problem of edema must be separated into two categories: generalized and localized.

Generalized edema is termed anasarca. In this condition, in addition to subcutaneous transudation, there may be transudation into serous cavities, resulting in ascites, pleural effusions, pericardial effusions, and other effects. Localized edema may occur with localized pathology. Systemic disease may, however, have local edema as a manifestation.

Causes of Generalized Edema	Excessive fluids, angioedema, congestive heart failure, cirrhosis, severe anemia, maternal diabetes, hemolytic disease, Henoch-Schönlein purpura, nephrotic syndrome, diabetes mellitus, kwashiorkor, beri beri, cystic fibrosis, protein-losing enteropathy, and galactosemia.
Causes of Localized Edema	Excessive crying, conjunctivitis, mumps, angioedema, insect bites, drugs, infectious mononucleosis, breech presentations, injections, sickle cell disease, mucocutaneous lymph node syndrome, congenital edema, Milroy's disease, trichinosis, congestive heart failure, filariasis, cavernous sinus thrombosis, and ethmoiditis.

Encopresis

Encopresis means fecal incontinence. The patient's history is most important in the formulation of a differential diagnosis. Specific points for questioning are: Is the patient toilet trained? What is the frequency of fecal soiling? At what time of day does the soiling occur? What is the stool character? What are the patient's urine and stool habits? Has the incontinence occurred recently, or has toilet training never been successful? Does defecation appear to be painful? Has there ever been any blood in the stools? Since the majority of patients suffering from encopresis have a psychological or emotional etiology for the soiling, complete psychological and developmental evaluations are essential in the diagnosis.

The objective portion of the examination should focus on the abdomen and the rectum. A complete neurological evaluation is also imperative.

Severe Constipation	Included under this heading are fecal impaction and painful defecation. Fecal impaction and soiling are frequently associated with severe psychological problems. Fecal soiling occurs when liquid stool spills around a solid fecal mass located low in the colon or rectum. The onset of soiling is usually after 3 years of age, and it occurs most commonly in males. Failure to thrive in these children is relatively uncommon. Defecation is frequently painful. There may be colicky abdominal pain. There may be palpable abdominal masses. On rectal examination, the ampulla is full of fecal material, a finding which is important in differentiating this kind of constipation from

Severe Constipation (cont'd)	Hirschsprung's disease, since, with the latter, the ampulla is usually empty. Abdominal distention is absent. Psychosocial evaluation may reveal contributing factors. Medical *and* psychological therapeutics are essential in management.
Mental Retardation	Mental retardation may be associated with fecal incontinence. Continence requires normal anatomical relationships, an intact voluntary and involuntary nervous system, and the awareness of the urge to defecate. Completing this cycle is the socialization of the individual and the child's ability to comprehend and control physiological urges.
Neurological Abnormalities	Neurological abnormalities, which may have fecal incontinence as an associated symptom, are spinal cord lesions, progressive degenerative diseases, spinal cord tumors, spinal cord trauma, and meningomyelocele. The neurological lesion is usually proximal to the second or third sacral nerve. Defecation is completely reflexive. The urge to defecate is absent. Denervation of the external sphincter occurs. There is an absence of sensation of rectal fullness and absence of function of the voluntary control over fecal continence.
Anal and Rectal Abnormalities	These may result in incontinence if the internal and external sphincter mechanisms are absent. If the levator ani and puborectalis muscles are present, continence can be achieved.

Cause of Encopresis

Cause of Encopresis	Constipation	Diarrhea	Hematochezia	Problems with Toilet Training	Abdominal Pain	Focal Neurological Signs	Lax Sphincter Tone	Urge to Defecate	Rectal Abnormalities
Emotional	4	3	0	4	3	0	0	0	0
Chronic constipation	4	2	2	2	3	0	4	0	0
Mental retardation	4	1	1	4	3	0–4	4	1–4	0
Neurological lesion	4	1	0	4	0	2	4	0	0–4
Anal/rectal abnormality	4	2	0	4	0	0	0	4	4

Epistaxis

Nosebleeds occur commonly in childhood, and can be a source of great anxiety to both children and their parents. Even the loss of a small amount of blood can appear to be a devastating blood loss to the anxious parent.

In the differential diagnosis of epistaxis, it is important to determine whether there has been trauma to the nose. It is equally important to determine whether the patient is a "nose picker." The volume of blood lost should be estimated, but it must be remembered that 5 cc of blood may look like a quart when the parent sees it on the child's face or pillow. It is important to determine whether the nosebleed stops spontaneously, as well as the amount of time taken for the bleeding to stop. A careful search of the history for other family members who have had similar problems gives the examiner a clue to genetically determined etiology. Earlier illness, easy bruisability, prior immunization, and prior rash must also be looked for in the history.

On physical examination, the site of active bleeding may not be readily apparent. The nose may be obstructed with "clots," which must be removed before a successful examination can be performed. The examiner should check under the patient's fingernails for the presence of dried blood. Other physical findings that should be noted are nasal deformities, bruises or petechiae, telangiectasias, nasal polyps, foreign bodies, nasal ulceration, and hypertension.

Epistaxis Digitorum (Nose Picking)	This is the most common cause of nosebleed in childhood. The site of trauma is usually the anterior nasal septum, and the bleeding may be unilateral or bilateral. Small excoriations may be seen on the nasal mucosa. The history may

Epistaxis Digitorum (Nose Picking) (cont'd)	be positive for nose picking. Dried blood may be present under the patient's fingernails. The remainder of the physical examination is normal.
Other Non-pathological Causes of Epistaxis	An environment with low humidity can cause the nasal mucosa to become dry and friable, resulting in minor nosebleeds. Vigorous nose blowing can also result in epistaxis. Upper respiratory tract infection can leave the nasal mucosa friable, and this, with a dry environment and frequent vigorous nose blowing, may result in epistaxis.
Foreign Body	Young children frequently insert foreign bodies into their noses and ears. A nasal foreign body should be suspected when there is a unilateral nasal obstruction, profuse foul nasal discharge, and recurrent epistaxis. The foreign body may be visualized during the physical examination. Removal may be extremely difficult and should be performed by an experienced physician under controlled conditions.
Trauma	Epistaxis is common following nasal trauma. The history may be positive for trauma. Mucosal lacerations, nasal bone fractures, and nasal deformities should alert the examiner to the possibility of trauma being the etiological factor for the epistaxis.
Nasal Polyposis	The mucosa overlying a nasal polyp is characteristically friable, and may bleed recurrently. The bleeding may be anterior or posterior. The history may be positive for allergy. Children with cystic fibrosis may present with nasal polyps. There may be signs and symptoms of nasal obstruction. Children with nasal polyposis are frequently mouth breathers. The polyps may be visualized on physical examination.

Hereditary Hemorrhagic Telangiectasia (HHT)	Hereditary hemorrhagic telangiectasia (HHT) is an uncommon illness. The most frequent presenting manifestation is epistaxis in childhood. There are superficial telangiectasias in the nasal mucosa. Telangiectasias may also be present on other mucous membranes, and are superficial and extremely friable. The spider-like lesions may be seen on the nasal mucosa. In older children, adolescents, and adults, the telangiectasias will appear in the skin, as well as the mucous membrane. The family history may be positive, in that other members of the family may have had nosebleeds as children or telangiectasias may have appeared on the skin during adulthood.
Blood Dyscrasias	Hematologic malignancies such as leukemia, as well as clotting disorders such as hemophilia and Christmas disease, are frequently associated with recurrent epistaxis. The bleeding may be profuse and difficult to stop. Other stigmata of blood dyscrasias, such as petechiae, purpura, easy bruisability, and hepatomegaly, splenomegaly, or both, may be present. Generalized lymphadenopathy may occur. There may be abnormal clotting profiles and abnormal platelet counts and platelet functions.
Other Illnesses Associated with Epistaxis	Pertussis, rubeola, hepatic disease, renal failure, syphilis, tuberculosis, hypertension, and hypervitaminosis.

Cause of Epistaxis

Cause of Epistaxis	History of Trauma	Family History	Easy Bruisability	Coagulation Profile Abnormality	Nasal Discharge	URI	Skin Lesions	Nasal Deformity	Hypertension
Self-induced trauma	4	0	0	0	0	0	0	4	0
Friable mucosa	2	0	0	0	1	0	0	2	0
Foreign body	1–4	0	0	0	4	0	0	4	0
Trauma	4	0	0	0	0	0	1–4	4	0
Polyps	0	4	0	0	4	0	0	4	0
HHT	0	2–4	0	0	0	0	1–4	0	0
Blood dyscrasia	0	1–4	4	1–4	0	0	3	0	0
Tumors	0	1	0	1	3	0	1	4	1
Hypertension	0	1	0	0	0	0	0	0	4

Failure to Thrive

The illnesses underlying failure to thrive range vastly in severity and prognosis. One of the most important aspects of diagnosis is to establish the fact that the child is not thriving, as opposed to being constitutionally small for his or her age. Failure to thrive describes children who are three standard deviations below the mean for weight (on a standard growth curve) and/or who show a persistent downward trend from their own established growth curve. The growth charts must be completed with at least three reference points. A child who begins in a percentile lower than the third percentile for the general pediatric population, but who maintains appropriate chronological growth velocity in that percentile, is not failing to thrive.

The causes of failure to thrive are multiple. It is important to differentiate between organic and nonorganic causes for the abnormal growth. A thorough history and physical examination will usually permit the examiner to distinguish between these two basic categories. Only in very rare instances will extensive laboratory evaluations be required.

Central nervous system disease and gastrointestinal disorders are the most common disorders associated with organic failure to thrive. Abnormalities of the genitourinary system and the endocrine system are also common causes.

| Nonorganic Failure to Thrive | This is the most common cause of failure to thrive. Approximately 70% of the patients will fall under this category. The etiology may be related to poverty (insufficient money available to provide sustenance for the child), accidents/errors in judgment by the caretaker in preparing food for the child (e.g., incorrect |

Nonorganic Failure to Thrive (cont'd)	reconstitution of formula, incorrect feeding techniques), or nutritional/caloric deprivation (the child receives inadequate nutrition because of a dysfunctional relationship between parent and child—the caretaker may be depressed, apathetic, and often overwhelmed).
Organic Failure to Thrive	Organic etiologies for failure to thrive occur in approximately 30% of the patients. Central nervous system disorders, gastrointestinal disorders, cardiovascular disorders, endocrine disorders, genetic abnormalities, and renal disorders should be considered in the evaluation. A comprehensive history and physical examination will usually provide sufficient clues to guide the evaluation of the patient.
Constitutional Short Stature	These children fall three standard deviations below the mean on a standard growth curve. They exhibit, however, no change in growth velocity and parallel their expected growth curve. A family history of short stature will usually be obtained.
Shifting Linear Growth	This refers to a genetic pattern of growth where the child (usually at 6 to 9 months of age) shifts his or her growth velocity to one of the parent's midgrowth channels.

Cause of Failure to Thrive	Weight < Third Percentile	Height < Third Percentile	Head Circumf. < Third Percentile	Poor Nutrition and Abnormal Diet History	Mother/Father Small	Low Growth/Changes in Velocity	Normal Growth Velocity	Diarrhea	Vomiting	Fevers	Recurrent Pneumonia	Recurrent Infections	Associated Physical Findings
Constitutional	0	4	0	0	4	0	0	0	0	0	0	0	0
Shifting linear growth	0	0	0	0	4	4	4	0	0	0	0	0	0
Maternal deprivation	4	2–4	0–4	4	0	4	0	0	0	0	0	0	0
CNS disease	4	3–4	2	2	0	4	0	*	*	0	0	0	4
Chronic illness	3	3	0	2	0	4	0	0	0	0	0	0	4
Malabsorption	4	2–4	0	1	0	4	0	4	1	0	0	0	1

Fever of Undetermined Etiology

Fever is a symptom associated with many disease processes and is one of the most common reasons for which the pediatrician is consulted. Most often the etiology is readily apparent (e.g., tonsillitis, otitis media, pneumonia); occasionally, the etiology is obscure and a high index of suspicion is necessary when formulating the differential diagnosis. Fever of unknown origin (FUO) is defined as an unremitting fever of greater than 101°F, lasting more than 2 weeks, for which no cause can be found clinically. It must be differentiated from fever of undetermined etiology, which is usually present for less than 2 weeks with no localizing signs or symptoms.

It is important to first document fever. When the parents state that fever is present, it is necessary to determine how the temperature was taken, the length of time the child has been febrile, and whether any medications had been given. Temperature curves may yield some clues to diagnosis; however, this is more reliable in adults than children. Any medication can alter the temperature curve.

The following differential diagnosis is aimed at those processes that may not be readily apparent. All causes of fever are not included.

Normal Variation	Fluctuation of body temperature throughout the day is normal. The range is relatively limited (97°F to 99°F). Rectal temperatures are generally one degree Fahrenheit higher than oral temperatures and two degrees higher than axillary. An oral temperature greater than 100°F (101°F rectal) is considered to be fever.

Malingering	This is infrequent in childhood. If malingering is suspected, temperature of voided urine can be used to obtain a true estimate of body core temperature. Urine temperature should approximate rectal temperature. A parent who regularly misrepresents fever in the child, which results in frequent invasive or painful diagnostic procedures may be manifesting symptoms of Munchausen's syndrome by proxy (a severe form of child maltreatment).
Infection	Fever is the most characteristic sign of infection. Unless the host is immunologically compromised and does not respond normally to infection, fever will often be present. The degree of temperature elevation is unreliable in distinguishing between viral, bacterial, fungal, and parasitic etiologies. The age of the patient is important. The significance of a temperature of 103°F varies between the neonate, the infant, the schoolage child, and the adolescent. A neonate with a temperature of 103°F should be considered septic until proven otherwise. An infant with the same temperature may look completely normal clinically, and the etiology may be a simple viral infection. The adolescent with fever will usually feel the effects at lower temperatures than the young child.
Meningitis	The signs and symptoms of meningeal infection are most commonly present in the older child and adolescent. Cephalgia, nuchal rigidity, and fever are frequent. In the infant, however, meningismus may be entirely absent. Kernig sign (inability to extend the legs when hips are flexed) and Brudzinski sign (flexion of the neck resulting in flexion of the hips, knees, or ankles) may be present, but these signs are unreliable in infants and children under 2 years of age. Nonspecific signs and symptoms, such

Meningitis (cont'd)	as irritability, lethargy, and poor feeding, are clues that the infant is sick. Convulsions may occur in children with meningeal infection, and may be the only presenting symptom. In general, an infant with fever and true irritability (with no obvious sign of infection) should be considered to have meningitis until proven otherwise. In meningitis, the spinal fluid will show a pleocytosis, decreased sugar content, and possibly bacteria on gram stain. Counterimmunoelectrophoresis and Limulus testing can give a rapid determination of etiology. It should be kept in mind that aseptic meningitis and tuberculous meningitis occur in childhood, and viral cultures and titers as well as acid-fast staining of the spinal fluid should be done if no apparent bacterial etiology can be found. Partially treated meningitis should also be considered if there is cerebrospinal fluid (CSF) pleocytosis and sterile cultures. Acridine orange stains may be helpful in partially treated patients. A careful history of medications given is necessary.
Other Intracranial Infections *Intracranial abscess*	Focal neurological signs and symptoms may be present.
Encephalitis	Seizures, personality changes, ataxia, and sensory changes may be present. Spinal fluid evaluation, CT scan, and nucleotide brain scan may assist in the diagnosis.
Urinary Tract Infection	Urinary tract symptoms such as dysuria, frequency, urgency, and incontinence are usually present in the older child and adolescent with urinary tract infection. These are subjective

Urinary Tract Infection (cont'd)	symptoms that are almost impossible to evaluate in the infant. Hematuria may occur, but otherwise these infants are seen only with the nonspecific symptoms of fever, poor feeding, vomiting, or diarrhea. The parents may report that the baby cries upon urination. The most important aspect of diagnosing urinary tract infection in the infant is a high index of suspicion. Urinalysis and culture are imperative. Pyuria and microscopic hematuria may signify infection. Suprapubic aspiration of urine may be necessary to avoid contamination of the specimen. Any culture positive for bacteria on a properly obtained urine specimen by suprapubic tap signifies infection.
Sepsis	Signs and symptoms of sepsis may be similar to those of meningitis. The fever is usually high and does not respond to antipyretic agents. The child may look overwhelmingly ill. Shock may be present. In the neonate, the temperature is more frequently very low. Hypothermia in the neonate is considered to result from sepsis until proven otherwise. A picture of metabolic acidosis may predominate. Blood cultures may yield the organism. Buffy coat smears stained with acridine orange may provide a rapid method for confirming the diagnosis (negative cultures and smears, however, do not rule out sepsis).
Suppurative Otitis Media	Suppurative otitis media is a frequent cause of fever in childhood. The history may reveal that the child has been pulling at the ear. There may be ear pain. The most reliable physical finding is loss of the normal tympanic membrane landmarks. Bulging of the membrane and loss of normal membrane compliance are characteristic of infection. Serous otitis media is characterized by membrane retraction and

Suppurative Otitis Media (cont'd)	air-fluid levels. Tympanic membrane color is extremely variable. A red drum does not mean infection; the color of the drum is determined by its vascularity and the source of illumination. Vigorous crying can engorge the tympanic membrane vessels and cause it to appear extremely red. The light reflex is also extremely variable, varying with the intensity of the illumination and the angle of the external canal.
Roseola Infantum	Roseola characteristically occurs in children 6 months to 4 years of age, with the greatest frequency being between 6 and 18 months. The temperature is high for 3 or 4 days. Children with roseola look remarkably well, even in the presence of a fever high enough to cause prostration. Posterior cervical and occipital adenopathy may be present. The pharynx may be slightly hyperemic. Leukopenia may be present during the febrile episode. On the third or fourth day the fever falls dramatically to normal. A diffuse maculopapular rash appears at the time of lysis of the fever or shortly thereafter.
Other Infections	Most childhood exanthems are ushered in by a variable prodromal period during which fever may occur; such conditions are rubeola, rubella, varicella, mumps, and erythema infectiosum. Other infections that are associated with fever are tuberculosis, appendicitis, bronchiolitis, hepatitis, osteomyelitis, pharyngitis, peritonsillar abscess, pneumonia, other viral syndromes, typhoid and paratyphoid fever, brucellosis, histoplasmosis, infectious mononucleosis, malaria, toxoplasmosis, cytomegalovirus, and walled-off abscess.

Dehydration	Cases of dehydration are often associated with fever; however, the etiology of the dehydration may be infectious and cause fever as part of the syndrome. Vomiting, diarrhea, and poor food and fluid intake may be reported in the history. Clinical signs of dehydration may be present, including poor skin turgor, sunken eyes, sunken fontanelles, dry mucous membranes, and oligouria/anuria. The degree of dehydration will determine the presenting signs and symptoms. Body fluid tonicity will determine the severity of symptoms. Clinical signs appear early and are more pronounced at lesser degrees of dehydration if the dehydration is hypotonic. Hypertonic dehydration may have few clinical signs and still be severe.
Absorption of Blood	Fever secondary to absorption of blood may occur postoperatively or following trauma. Subdural hematoma, mediastinal hematoma, hemothorax, and hemoperitoneum may be associated with fever. It must be kept in mind that even though a resolving hematoma may cause fever, infection may be present as well; therefore, appropriate cultures must be obtained.
Aspirin	In contrast to their antipyretic effect at therapeutic levels, salicylates in overdose cause fever. A careful history is necessary. Other signs and symptoms of salicylism are elevated salicylate levels, positive ferric chloride test, tinnitus, tachypnea, hyperpnea ("panting dog" breathing), alkalosis, acidosis, and hypoglycemia.
Malignancy	The common presenting signs and symptoms of malignancy in adults are notoriously absent in children. Hematologic malignancies as well

Malignancy (cont'd)	as solid tumors frequently present as fevers of unknown etiology. A high index of suspicion is necessary for correct diagnosis.
Other Causes of Fever with No Readily Apparent Etiology	Rheumatoid arthritis, systemic lupus erythematosus, periarteritis nodosa, drugs and poisons, ulcerative colitis, Crohn's disease, ectodermal dysplasia, Caffey's disease, agammaglobulinemia, familial dysautonomia, and sickle cell anemia.

Cause of Fever of Undetermined Etiology	Type of Fever	Signs of Dehydration	CBC Abnormalities	Tachypnea	Tachycardia	CSF Pleocytosis	Urinalysis Abnormalities	Decreased Complement	Joint Pain/Swelling	Rash	Meningeal Signs	Anemia	Leukopenia	Leukocytosis
Normal variation	(4)	0	0	0	0	0	0	0	0	0	0	0	0	0
Occult infection	4	0	3	0–1	3	2	0–2	1	1	1	2	1–2	1–2	2
Dehydration	0	4	3	4	4	0	3	0	0	0	0	0	1	3
Malignancy	0	0	1–4	1	1	1	1–2	0	0	0–1	0–1	0–4	2–4	2–4
Collagen-vascular disease (JRA)	2–4	0	4	1	3	0	0	0	4	1	0	4	1	2
Collagen-vascular disease (SLE)	2	0	4	1	3	0	3	2–4	4	1	0	3	2	0
Drugs	2	0	0	1	0	0	0	0	0	2	0	0	0	0

Frequency of Urination

Urinary frequency is defined as an increase in the number of voids per day. It does not refer to urine volume, since sensation of the need to void may be present, but the volume of urine produced is small. The history should be searched for the presence of other symptoms referable to the urinary tract.

Urinary Tract Infection	Urinary frequency is one of the more common symptoms associated with urinary tract infection in childhood. Other associated symptoms may be dysuria, urgency, hesitancy, dribbling, incontinence, and hematuria.
Large Fluid Intake	The intake of large amounts of fluid will result in urinary frequency. There are usually no other symptoms. The volume of urine produced is large (polyuria).
Diabetes Mellitus	Polyuria, polydipsia, and polyphagia are the classic triad of diabetes mellitus. The presenting signs and symptoms may be related to ketoacidosis, but the history will usually be positive for the triad.
Posterior Urethral Valves	In children with posterior urethral valves, the volume of urine is small, and there may be a sensation of incomplete emptying. Dribbling and hematuria may occur. The bladder may be palpable. Hydronephrosis may be present.
Other Causes of Frequency of Urination	Nephritis, appendicitis, drugs, renal failure, adrenal cortical hyperplasia, and meatal stenosis.

Cause of Frequency of Urination	Urgency	Dysuria	Hematuria	Pyesis	Glucosuria	Hyposthenuria	Hyperthenuria	Incontinence	Polyuria	Polyphagia	Polydipsia	Anorexia
Increased fluid intake	1	0	0	0	0	4	0	0	4	0	0	0
UTI	3	3	3	3	0	1	0	1	0	3	0	0
Diabetes mellitus	0	0	0	0	4	0	4	0	4	4	4	0
Diabetes insipidus	1	0	0	0	0	4	0	0	4	0	4	3
Distal UT obstruction	2	0	1	1	0	2	0	2	0	0	0	0

Gingivitis/Stomatitis

Inflammation, infection, or both, of the oral mucosa is an extremely distressing symptom. It may present as an isolated inflammation or infection, or may be a manifestation of systemic illness.

When investigating the patient's history, special attention should be paid to the following questions: Are there any undercurrent illnesses? When was the patient's last dental visit? Has the patient taken any drugs or medications? Is there a history of diabetes? Does the patient have seizures? What constitutes the patient's diet? Is there a history of trauma?

The physical examination should focus on the following: Mouth, pharynx, and teeth: Are they in good repair? Is there involvement of the anterior (oral) or posterior (pharyngeal) mucosa, or gingivae? Teeth: What is the state of repair of the teeth? Is the patient a mouth breather? Lymph nodes: Is there localized or generalized adenopathy? Neurological examination: Are there focal or generalized neurological abnormalities? Are there other signs of vitamin deficiency? Lacrimal and parotid glands: Are there signs and symptoms of exocrine glandular dysfunction?

| **Infection**
Herpes gingivostomatitis | The lesions of herpes gingivostomatitis are small, whitish-yellow, shallow ulcerations, and are very painful. They are usually located on the anterior buccal mucosa, but may occur anywhere in the mouth and pharynx. If the lesions are located at the vermilion border of the lip, crusting may occur. The temperature is high and may be elevated 1 to 3 days prior to eruption of lesions. |

Coxsackie virus	The lesions of Coxsackie virus infection appear as very small, shallow, yellowish ulcerations. They appear most commonly on the posterior buccal and pharyngeal mucosa, especially the anterior tonsillar pillars, and are usually quite painful.
Vincent angina	Vincent angina is a mixed infection of the oral mucosa. It usually occurs in ill or debilitated children. There is a fetid odor associated with Vincent stomatitis.
Thrush	Oral monilial infections appear as irregular white plaques on the oral mucosa; their removal is difficult, and the underlying tissue is friable and bleeds with removal of the plaque.
Allergic Reactions	Multiple mucous membranes may be involved in allergic reactions. The lesions may vary from aphthous ulcerations to bullae formation. The mucosa may be friable, and there may be diffuse swelling. There may or may not be similar cutaneous manifestations.
Aphthous Ulcers	Aphthous ulcers, or canker sores, are small, recurrent, whitish ulcers that are quite painful but not associated with systemic illness. They may occur anywhere on the oral mucosa, but tend to localize anteriorly.
Drugs	Reactions of the oral mucosa to drugs are similar to its allergic reactions. With phenytoin there are varying degrees of gingival hyperplasia. The mucosa is friable and bleeds easily. There is usually a history of seizures.
Stevens-Johnson Syndrome	This is a hypersensitive disorder, characterized by skin and mucous membrane lesions. The cutaneous lesions are variable and range from maculourticarial to bullous. The characteristic iris lesion is an erythematous patch, with a dusky center and red, raised borders.

Stevens-Johnson Syndrome (cont'd)	The mucosal lesions are superficial ulcerations and may be the only manifestation.
Vitamin Deficiency *Riboflavin deficiency*	Riboflavin deficiency is manifested by cheilosis (cracking and ulceration of the angle of the mouth), glossitis, keratitis, conjunctivitis, photophobia, lacrimation, neovascularization of the cornea, and seborrheic dermatitis. There is low excretion of riboflavin in the urine.
Niacin deficiency	In niacin deficiency there are, characteristically, glossitis (redness and swelling of the tip of the tongue), stomatitis, dermatitis (sunburn-like rash on the face, neck and hands), diarrhea, and dementia.
Vitamin B_6 deficiency	Peripheral neuropathy, cheilosis, glossitis, and seborrheic dermatitis point toward pyridoxine deficiency. Convulsions are common in infancy. Anemia (microcytichypochromic) is also present. Tryptophane challenge is diagnostic.
Scurvy	Scurvy is marked by a bluish-purple, spongy swelling of the gums, especially in the region of the upper incisors. Other characteristic symptoms include irritability, leg pain (causing a pseudoparalysis), subperiosteal hemorrhage, petechiae, fever, anemia, follicular hyperkeratosis, and delayed wound healing.
Dental Abnormalities *Carious teeth*	Dental infections may be associated with contiguous gingival infection and inflammation.
Malocclusion	In malocclusion, chronic irritation of the mucosa can cause inflammation of the gingival mucosa in the areas of malformation.

Mouth Breathing	Chronic mouth breathing causes dryness of the oral mucosa; this dry mucosa is friable and will bleed easily on contact. The tongue and palate are involved, as well as the gingivae. The tongue may become furrowed.

Hematemesis

Hematemesis is a relatively uncommon problem during infancy and childhood. Its presence should alert the physician to look for potentially life-threatening conditions. A large amount of blood may be lost rapidly into the gastrointestinal tract before being noticed. Hemoglobin is irritating to the gastrointestinal tract and may cause vomiting and mass peristaltic movements.

It is important to question the parents about food and drink recently ingested. Red colored food or drink may look like blood to the parents.

Determine the volume of blood in the vomitus. Blood streaking has different significance than the vomiting of frank blood. Question the parents about previous recent illnesses, ingestion of drugs or foreign objects, coughing, nosebleeds, and bleeding tendencies.

Newborn Period *Swallowed maternal blood*	The Apt test differentiates maternal from fetal blood; fetal hemoglobin resists denaturation by sodium hydroxide. Mix a small amount of stool or vomitus with tap water (one part sample to five parts water) and centrifuge. Add 1 cc of 0.25 N NaOH to the supernatant. Observe the color after 5 minutes. Adult hemoglobin will turn brownish-yellow. Fetal hemoglobin will remain pink.
Hemorrhagic disease of the newborn	In neonatal hemorrhagic disease there are commonly other signs and symptoms of a bleeding diathesis; there are petechiae, ecchymosis, purpura, and hematochezia. There will be marked decrease in the vitamin K-dependent clotting factors prothrombin and factors VII, IX, and X.

Necrotizing enterocolitis	Infants with this condition are extremely ill looking. Necrotizing enterocolitis occurs most commonly in artificially fed premature newborns. There are abdominal distention, hematochezia, diarrhea/purulent stools, and frequently shock. Thrombocytopenia also occurs. Pneumatosis intestinalis and air in the hepatic portal system on X-ray examination of the abdomen are diagnostic.
Other causes of hematemesis in the newborn	Stress ulcer, hemorrhagic gastritis, trauma secondary to nasogastric tube, neonatal hepatic necrosis, duplications, and hiatal hernia.
Any Age Group *Swallowed blood*	The source of bleeding may be from the nose, throat, or teeth. Overt bleeding may not be readily apparent, and a careful history and physical examination is of the utmost importance. The vomitus usually contains frank blood if from epistaxis. Oozing from the gingivae or pharynx will usually cause blood-streaked vomitus. Blood in the stomach for extended periods of time will resemble coffee grounds.
Protracted vomiting	The source of bleeding secondary to protracted vomiting may be irritation of the pharynx or esophagus. Mallory-Weiss syndrome is exceedingly rare in childhood.
Peptic ulcer disease	The volume of blood vomited is usually large. The patient may not look sick. There are usually associated anemia and abdominal pain, which may be relieved by eating. Cushing ulcers are usually associated with overwhelming infection. Curling ulcers are usually associated with thermal injury. Diagnosis is made by upper gastrointestinal series and endoscopy.

Erosive gastritis/esophagitis	The vomitus is usually blood streaked. There are associated pain and dysphagia. There may be a history of ingestion of a strong acid, alkali, or aspirin.
Esophagitis	The volume of blood is small. There are also dysphagia and failure to thrive. The source may be hiatal hernia or severe chalasia. The diagnosis may be made by esophagogram or endoscopy.
Gastric outlet obstruction	Pyloric stenosis, webs or diaphragms, and scarring.
Esophageal varices	Signs and symptoms of portal hypertension. The volume of blood vomited is usually large.
Foreign body	History of ingestion of a foreign body (nail, pin, etc.), and eating foods which contain bones. The foreign body or bone may or may not be seen on plain X-ray film of the abdomen, chest, or neck.
Other causes of hematemesis	Hemangioma, telangiectasia, tumor, and blood dyscrasia.

Cause of Hematemesis

Cause of Hematemesis	Petechiae/Purpura	Hemotochezia	Abdominal Distention	Abnormal Clotting	Nose Bleeds	Nonbloody Vomiting	Abdominal Pain	Skin Color Change and Pallor	Oral Lesions	Volume of Blood	Hepatomegaly	Splenomegaly	Laboratory Study of Emesis
Swallowed blood	0	0	0	0	3	0	0	0	0–3	0	0	0	4
Hemorrhagic disease of newborn	3	0	0	4	1	1	0	3	0	3	0	0	0
Ingestion	1	0	0	1	0	1	1	2	2	0	2	0	2
NEC	2	2	4	3	0	1	3	3	0	2	2	2	0
Protracted vomiting	0	0	0	0	0	3	2	0	0	1	0	0	0
Peptic ulcer	0	1	1	0	0	1	4	0	0	3	0	0	0
Esophagitis	0	0	0	0	0	3	1	0	0	0	0	0	0
Gastritis	0	0	1	0	0	2	4	0	0	0	0	0	0
Obstruction	0	0	4	0	0	3	4	0	0	1	0	0	0
Varices	3	0	1	3	1	0	2	3	0	4	3	3	0
Foreign body	0	0	1	0	3	2	2	0	0	1	0	0	1
Blood dyscrasia	3	0	0	4	2	0	0	2	2	2	2	2	0

Hematuria

Hematuria is the excretion of bloody urine. The blood may appear on gross examination or may appear microscopically. If blood is grossly present, the color of the urine may range from bright red to dark brown. The etiology may be localized to the lower urinary tract, may originate in the upper urinary tract, or may be a renal manifestation of a systemic disease process.

The history should focus on the following: Generalized factors: Is the patient taking any medications or drugs? Are there any allergies? Does the patient or family member have a known bleeding disorder? Is there abdominal or back pain? Local factors: Has there been any recent trauma? Does the patient masturbate? Could the patient have inserted a foreign object into the urethra? Infection: Is there associated dysuria, frequency, urgency, polyuria, or incontinence? Has there been a fever or recent systemic infection?

The perineum and urethral meatus should be thoroughly inspected. The presence of blood should be documented qualitatively with dipstick testing and quantitatively by microscopic methods. Intravenous pyelogram (IVP), voiding cystourethrogram (VCU), and cystoscopy may be useful in establishing a diagnosis.

Urinary Tract Infection	Infection in any region of the urinary tract may result in hematuria. Urinary frequency, urgency, hesitancy, dribbling, dysuria, fever, and incontinence may be present. If the upper urinary tract is involved, costovertebral angle pain, hypertension, and nephrotic syndrome may occur.

Urethritis/ Urethral Caruncle	Dysuria is frequently present. Hesitancy may occur. The blood is bright red and small in volume. There is usually an absence of systemic symptoms.
Meatal Ulceration	Symptoms are similar to those of urethritis and urethral caruncles. The ulceration may be visualized. Diaper rash or balantitis may be present.
Foreign Body	Insertion of a foreign body can cause hematuria, dysuria, urethral obstruction, and a foul-smelling, purulent discharge.
Calculi	The volume of blood may be large. Renal colic and other urinary tract symptoms may occur.
Trauma	The history may be positive for trauma. The perineum may be involved. Child abuse should be suspected when there is trauma to the perineum.
Posterior Urethral Valves	Dribbling, incomplete bladder emptying, hematuria, and hydronephrosis may occur. The bladder and other abdominal masses (hydroureter) may be palpable. There may be hypertension.
Glomerulonephritis	Hematuria is common. Red blood cell casts are usually seen in the urinary sediment. There may be a history of prior streptococcal infection. Fever and hypertension may occur.
Other Causes of Hematuria	Immunoglobulin A (IgA) nephropathy, benign familial hematuria, hydronephrosis, schistosomiasis, telangiectasia, blood dyscrasia, Henoch-Schönlein purpura, renal vein thrombosis, and subacute bacterial endocarditis.

Cause of Hematuria

Cause of Hematuria	Abdominal Pain	Flank Pain	Dysuria	Polyuria	Frequency	Urgency	Dribbling or Incontinence	Fever	Pyuria	Elevated Blood Pressure	Decreased Complement	Abnormal IVP
Cystitis	3	0	4	0	4	4	3	2	4	0	0	0
Urethritis	0	0	4	0	4	4	1	1	4	0	0	0
Pyelonephritis	1	3	1	0	0	0	0	3	4	2	0	1–4
Glomerulonephritis	1	2	1	0	0	0	0	1	3	4	1–4	1–4
Meatal ulceration	0	0	4	0	4	4	1	0	4	0	0	0
Foreign body (urethral)	0	0	2	0	1	0–4	0	0	2	0	0	0
Trauma	1	2	0	0	1	0–4	0	0	2	0–4	0	*
Calculi	3	3	0	0	1	1	0	0	2		0	4
Posterior urethral valves	0	0	0	0	1	1	2	0	0	1	0	2
Henoch-Schönlein purpura	3	0	0	0	0	0	0	2	1	1	0	0
Stevens-Johnson syndrome	0	0	1	0	0	1	0	4	2	0	0	0
IgA nephropathy	1	1	0	0	0	0	0	0	0	1	0	0
Subacute bacterial endocarditis	0	0	0	0	0	0	0	0	2	0	1	0
Renal vein thrombosis	1	1	0	0	(4)	0	0	0	2	0–4	0	4
Blood dyscrasia	0	0	0	0	0	0	0	0	0	0	0	0

Hemoptysis

Hemoptysis and hematemesis are frequently difficult to differentiate. When evaluating a patient with hemoptysis, the differential diagnosis of hematemesis should also be considered. Children infrequently expectorate sputum; therefore, the bloody sputum may not be evident until the patient vomits.

Significant historical information is as follows: Description of the episode: Was the patient coughing or vomiting prior to the episode? Has there been a recent nosebleed? Description of the sputum: Was the sputum streaked or speckled with blood? Was the sputum totally red? Was the color of the blood bright red, dark, or rusty? Medications: Has the patient been taking any medications? Associated questions: Has there been chest pain, vomiting, fever, or easy bruising? Are the patient's immunizations up to date? Could there have been aspiration of a foreign body?

Physical examination should focus on the chest, mouth, and pharynx. Are the breath sounds equal? Are there rales or adventitious sounds? Is there evidence of trauma? Are there nasal, pharyngeal, or oral lesions? Is there evidence of ecchymosis or petechiae?

Common Causes of Hemoptysis	Protracted cough, epistaxis, pneumonia, foreign body, and vomiting.
Less Common Causes of Hemoptysis	Blood dyscrasia, tumor, telangiectasia, bronchiectasis, congestive heart failure, uremia, pulmonary abcess, hemosiderosis, and trauma.

Cause of Hemoptysis	Color	Vomiting	Pain	Epistaxis	Increased Blood Volume	Trauma	Foreign Body	Bruisability	Oral/Nasal Lesions	Unequal Breath Sounds
Pneumonia/bronchiectasis	4	1	1	0	2	0	0	0	0	1
Protracted cough	0	1	1	0	1	0	2	0	0	0
Foreign body	2	0	1	1	0	0	4	0	1	3
Trauma	0	0	3	2	0–4	4	0	0	1	4
Telangiectasia	0	0	0	3	2	0	0	0	4	0
Blood dyscrasia	0	0	0	3	4	0	0	4	2	2
Tumors	0	0	0	0	0–4	0	0	0	1	3

Hypoglycemia

Hypoglycemia is not an uncommon symptom during infancy and childhood. It occurs with a frequency of 2 to 3 per 1,000 live births in neonates. Symptoms in the small infant may be absent or may include irritibility, poor feeding, tremors, convulsions, apnea, cyanosis, hypotonia, high-pitched cry, and difficulty in maintaining body temperature. Older children may experience weakness, pallor, diaphoresis, tachycardia, tremors, abnormal behavior, lethargy, and/or seizures. If the hypoglycemia is secondary to an underlying disease process, signs and symptoms may be related to the disease.

Neonatal	Neonatal hypoglycemia is defined as blood sugar less than 30 mg/dl in the term newborn or less than 20 mg/dl in the preterm newborn (in the first 72 hours after birth). Blood sugar below these levels requires treatment, even in the absence of symptoms. If symptoms are present, the blood sugar concentration should be correlated with the clinical condition when determined if treatment is necessary.
	Causes of neonatal hypoglycemia include neisidioblastosis, small for gestational age, infants of diabetic mothers, septicemia, hypoxia, maternal drugs (oral hypoglycemic agents, beta-adrenergic agonists and antagonists) and galactosemia.
Ketotic Hypo-glycemia	This is the most common cause of hypoglycemia in childhood. It occurs in children between the ages of 18 months and 5 years. There is usually spontaneous remission by 9 to 10 years of age. Males are more commonly affected. It

Ketotic Hypo-glycemia (cont'd)	is characterized by episodic *symptomatic* hypoglycemia and ketonemia. The attacks are usually related to periods of fasting (occurring most often in the morning hours), illness or vomiting. The symptomatic attack may be precipitated 8 to 16 hours after initiation of a hypocaloric ketogenic diet. Between attacks, the glucose tolerance tests are normal.
Drug Ingestion	Drug-induced hypoglycemia may be caused by the ingestion of ethyl alcohol, salicylates, acetaminophen, and oral hypoglycemic agents.
Insulin Overdosage	A history of insulin-dependent diabetes mellitus in a patient with hypoglycemia or in a family member may suggest excessive insulin administration.
Reye's Syndrome	Vomiting, hepatomegaly, behavior changes, coma, elevated liver function tests, hyperammonemia, and profound hypoglycemia are characteristic of Reye's syndrome.
Galactosemia	Hepatomegaly and jaundice are frequently present. Weight loss, lethargy, hypotonia, and severe infections are common.
Other Causes of Hypoglycemia	Neisidioblastosis, adrenal insufficiency, glycogen storage disease, fructose–1,6–diphosphatase deficiency, and hereditary fructose intolerance.

Hypotonia

Hypotonia is a state of decreased muscle tone, at times associated with weakness. It may be discovered at birth (congenital) or may be acquired later in childhood. The abnormality may lie in the central nervous system (CNS), peripheral nervous system (PNS), or end organ (muscles). Signs and symptoms vary according to the location of the abnormality. Signs and symptoms that suggest hypotonia are hypermobile or extensible joints, persistence of head lag after the third month of life, lack of head control, and slipping of the patient through the examiner's hands when held suspended by the axillae. Paucity of intrauterine movements, difficulty swallowing or sucking, and limited activity when left unattended should alert the examiner to the possibility of hypotonia. The location may be differentiated by checking the patient's reflexes: CNS disorders are characterized by brisk reflexes and a positive Babinski sign, while reflexes are usually weak or absent in PNS disorders.

Werdnig-Hoffman Disease (Infantile Spinal Muscle Atrophy)	There are marked hypotonia and weakness, especially of the proximal muscle groups. Deep tendon reflexes are absent and fasciculations of the tongue may be noted when the baby is at rest (not crying). The sensory system is normal. There may be associated pectus excavatum. Aspiration pneumonia is common.
	Four types of Werdnig-Hoffman disease have been described. *Type 1* is characterized by the onset at less than 3 months of age of hypotonia and weakness. The baby has a feeble cry, sucks poorly, and has poor activity when at rest. The joints may appear hypermobile. *Type 2* is characterized by an onset between 3

Werdnig-Hoffman Disease *(Infantile Spinal Muscle Atrophy)* (cont'd)	months and 1 year of age. There is delayed motor development. The patients can usually roll from side to side, but rarely are able to sit without support. Resting tremors of the fingers may be present. *Type 3* disease has its onset between 1 and 2 years of age. There is delayed muscle development and the patients usually sit without support. They rarely walk without assistance, and there is marked proximal muscle weakness. *Type 4* disease has its onset between 2 and 5 years of age. There is extreme proximal muscle weakness and the patient's presentation may mimic Duchenne's muscular dystrophy.
Benign Congenital Hypotonia	There are generalized weakness, limpness, and hypotonia at birth, which characteristically improve with age. Sitting and standing may be delayed. The deep tendon reflexes are variable and respirations are rarely affected.
Birth Trauma	Most children who suffer cerebral damage from birth trauma (spastic or flaccid paralysis) initially present with hypotonia. Spasticity occurs with time. The patient's history may reveal a complicated gestation, labor, and/or delivery.
Congenital Malformations	Congenital malformations of the CNS may be associated with hypotonia. Other characteristics may be readily apparent at birth (e.g., anencephaly, encephalocele) or may appear later in infancy. The serial measurement of the child's head circumference may be helpful in identifying hydrocephalus or microcephaly. Transillumination of the skull may reveal useful information.
Maternal Drugs	There may be a history of drug use/abuse by the mother. Hypotonia and respiratory depression occur when the mother has taken or re-

Maternal Drugs (cont'd)	ceived the drug close to the time of delivery. Chronic drug abuse may result in neonatal narcotic withdrawal syndrome. Narcotic analgesics used during labor may cause hypotonia in the newborn. Generalized CNS depression and respiratory depression may occur.
Intoxications	Insecticides (especially organophosphates) may induce hypotonia. Clinical features simulate a myasthenic crisis with weakness, bulbar involvement, difficulty in handling secretions, and respiratory distress.
Infantile Botulism	This results from ingestion of the spores and the enteral production of toxin. It usually occurs in children younger than 1 year of age. There is often a history of honey ingestion. Constipation is usually the first presenting symptom. A weak cry, poor suck, difficulty in handling secretions, hypotonia and weakness, head lag, and poor respiratory excursions are concomitant symptoms.
Poliomyelitis	Development of asymmetric flaccid weakness of the muscles, preceded by a mild upper respiratory tract or gastrointestinal tract infection may suggest polio. If the cranial nerves are involved, abnormalities in sucking and swallowing and hoarseness and stridor can occur.
Guillain-Barré Syndrome	Distal muscle weakness and pain occurs, usually preceded 1 to 3 weeks by an upper respiratory tract or gastrointestinal tract infection. The weakness may ascend and involve the muscles of respiration. Difficulty in swallowing signifies bulbar involvement. Deep tendon reflexes are markedly decreased or absent. There is often spontaneous remission in 4 to 6 weeks. There is usually a marked elevation in the protein content of the cerebrospinal fluid (without pleocytosis). Electromyography re-

Guillain-Barré Syndrome (cont'd)	veals neuropathic changes and fibrillation potentials.
Muscular Dystrophy	The onset of symptoms in the Duchenne's type (most common) is usually between 3 and 6 years of age. There are clumsiness and falling. Pseudohypertrophy of the gastrocnemius and deltoid muscles occurs. There is progressive proximal muscle weakness of the shoulder and pelvic girdles. Most patients have difficulty on standing from a supine position (Gowers' sign), toe walking, and climbing stairs. Deep tendon reflexes are usually absent. The creatine phosphokinase level is markedly elevated.
Myasthenia Gravis	Bulbar weakness occurs in association with ophthalmoplegia, ptosis, expressionless facies, weak suck and swallow, weak cry, and respiratory distress. There are generalized muscle weakness after inactivity, lack of movement, a weak grasp reflex, poor Moro reflex, and a poor rooting reflex. Deep tendon reflexes are usually present. There are three forms of myasthenia gravis: *transient neonatal* (onset is within the first 24 hours of life, the mother is myasthenic, and the symptoms resolve in 3 to 6 weeks), *congenital* (onset is usually later in infancy and the symptoms do not resolve), and *juvenile* (onset is between 5 and 10 years of age). Diagnosis is confirmed using a Tensilon® test.
Other Causes of Hypotonia	Down's syndrome, hyperthyroidism, hypercalcemia, glycogen storage diseases, ricketts, trauma to the spinal cord, spinal cord tumor, intracranial abscess or tumor, lipoidosis, Prader-Willi syndrome, Marfan's syndrome, Ehlers-Danlos syndrome, arthrogryposis congenita, congenital myopathies, dermatomyosi-

Other Causes of Hypotonia (cont'd)	tis, paramyotonia congenita, periodic familial paralysis, hypoxia, and familial dysautonomia.

Cause of Hypotonia	Asymmetrical	Generalized	Umbilical Hernia	Prolonged Jaundice	Weak Cry	Head Lag	Regression	Abnormal Facies	Lid Lag	Fever	Weak Suck	Large Tongue	Cataracts
Hypothyroidism	0	4	3	3	3	3	0	2	3	0	2	4	0
Hypercalcemia	0	3	0	3	1	0	4	1	0	0	1	0	3
Guillain-Barré syndrome	0	2	0	0	0–4	0–4	4	0	0	0	0–4	0	0
Cerebral palsy	0–4	0–4	0	0	0–4	0–4	0	0–4	0	0	0–4	0	0
Down's syndrome	0	4	1	1	0	3	0	4	0	0	0	4	1
Tumor	3	1	0	0	1	1	4	0	1	0	1	0	0
Myasthenia gravis	0	4	0	0	2	*	0	0	2	0	2	0	0
Werdnig-Hoffman disease	0	3	0	0	1	3	1	0	0	0	2	0	0
Glycogen storage disease	2	2	0	0	1	1	2	1	0	0	1	0	0
Dysautonomia	1	0	0	0	0	0	4	0	0	4	3	0	0
Prader-Willi syndrome	0	4	0	0	3	4	0	4	0	0	3	0	0
Ehlers-Danlos syndrome	0	2	0	0	0	0	0	2	0	0	0	0	0
Amyotonia congenital	2	2	0	0	0	0	1	0	0	0	3	0	0

Irritability

Irritability is generally defined as an immoderate reaction to a stimulus. The clinical connotation is "excessive or exaggerated crying or fretfulness." The child is unable to be soothed.

Parents frequently describe their children as being irritable when waking for frequent nighttime feedings or when their diapers are wet or soiled. This crankiness must be differentiated from true irritability. The truly irritable child cannot be soothed by being held, fed or having his or her diaper changed. On the contrary, crying and screaming are often exacerbated if the child is disturbed. The irritable child will usually refuse feedings.

Meningitis/ Sepsis	In the neonatal period and infancy, *true* irritability means meningitis or sepsis, until proven otherwise. The child cannot be soothed. The cry is usually high-pitched and shrill. Fever or hypothermia may be present. Meningeal signs may be completely absent. Feeding is poor. Vomiting may occur. There may be alternating lethargy.
Other Infectious Causes of Irritability	Urinary tract infection, otitis media, gastroenteritis, and pneumonia.
Narcotic Withdrawal Syndrome	This is seen in infants born to narcotic-addicted mothers. The infant is irritable, tremulous, sneezes frequently, and coughs. Drooling is increased, and constipation or diarrhea may occur. The infant is most commonly small for gestational age, and is frequently born prematurely.

Teething	Irritability can be caused by simple teething. There is an increase in the amount of drooling. The gums may be red or swollen. The sharp edge of the teeth, cutting through the gums, may be palpated.
Colic	Colic occurs early in infancy. It is characterized by intermittent acute abdominal pain, where the infant has a shrill cry, may sweat profusely, and may draw his or her legs up to the chest. The colic is paroxysmal. The child is otherwise healthy.
Other Causes of Irritability	Hunger, food intolerance, psychological problems, lack of sleep, and drug reactions (phenobarbital, antihistamines).

Cause of Irritability	Fever	Hypothermia	Lethargy	Meningismus	Maternal Drugs	Tremors	Sneezing	Drooling	Persistent	Intermittent	Medication/Drugs	Abnormal Spinal Fluid	Frequency (Urinary)	Dysuria	Pyuria	Abnormal Tympanic Membrane
Meningitis	4	0	3	3	0	0	0	0	4	0	0	4	0	0	0	0
Septicemia	3	1	3	0	0	0	0	0	3	2	0	1	0	0	0	0
UTI	3	0	0	0	0	0	0	0	0	3	0	0	1	2	4	0
Narcotic withdrawal	0	0	1	0	4	4	4	3	3	3	0	0	0	0	0	0
Teething pain	2	0	0	0	0	0	0	3	1	3	0	0	0	0	0	0
Colic	0	0	0	0	0	1	0	0	0	4	0	0	0	0	0	0
Drugs	0	0	3	0	0	0	0	0	2	2	4	0	0	0	0	0
Lack of sleep	0	0	4	0	0	0	0	0	2	2	0	0	0	0	0	0
Otitis media	4	0	0	0	0	0	0	0	1–3	1–3	0	0	0	0	0	4

Joint Pain

Painful joints may be a manifestation of local or systemic illness. It is important to determine whether the patient is complaining of arthralgia or arthritis. It is also important to determine the number of joints involved, whether the pain has migrated from one joint to another, whether the small, nonweight-bearing joints or large, weight-bearing joints are involved, the presence of joint effusion, whether there is limitation of motion of the joints involved, whether any drugs have been ingested, and whether there are other systemic manifestations of illness.

Joint pain in infants is difficult to assess. There may be crying or screaming upon movement of the joint. The extremity is usually held still, since movement may increase the pain.

Trauma	The history may be positive for injury to the joint. Deformity, swelling, discoloration, and limitation of motion may be present. Effusion or hemarthrosis may occur. The pain is usually increased by motion or weight bearing.
Infection *Septic* *arthritis*	The most common age for septic arthritis is 6 months or younger, but it may occur at any age. Septic arthritis may be secondary to hematogenous spread, direct extension, or direct inoculation. The onset is acute. In younger patients, signs of septicemia may predominate. Fever is usually present along with systemic signs of toxicity. In older patients, systemic toxicity may be absent. Fever may occur later in the course of the illness. The larger joints are more commonly involved. The joint is swollen and tender, and there is pain with

Infection *Septic arthritis* (cont'd)	motion. If the hip is involved, dislocation may occur.
Osteomyelitis	Osteomyelitis may mimic septic arthritis and the two entities may be difficult to differentiate on clinical grounds. With osteomyelitis, however, a careful physical examination may reveal that the suspected joint may be passively mobilized without pain.
Sickle Cell Anemia	Joint pain is common in sickle cell disease and is characteristic of vasoocclusive crisis. The first symptoms appear after 1 year of age. The hand-foot syndrome is caused by infarction of the small bones of the hands. Swelling of the hands, the feet, or both is bilaterally symmetrical. In older patients, there is swelling and pain of the large joints.
Serum Sickness	This is an allergic type of reaction. Symptoms appear from 1 to 2 weeks following the administration of the antigenic material. Generalized urticaria, pruritis, fever, lymphadenopathy, myalgia, arthralgia, and arthritis may all occur.
Henoch-Schönlein Purpura	There is acute or gradual onset of malaise and fever. Skin lesions occur in all patients; the lesions are variable and usually occur on the lower extremities. Arthritis occurs in 67% of patients, with the large joints being involved. The joints are swollen, tender, and painful, and effusions are frequently present. Gastrointestinal and renal symptoms may occur.
Collagen Diseases *Systemic lupus erythematosus (SLE)*	Arthralgia is a common manifestation of SLE. The joints may become stiff. There may be no physical signs, but, occasionally, the joints are swollen and warm. Fever is common. Malaise may occur. A rash that occurs over the malar

Collagen Diseases *Systemic lupus erythematosus (SLE)* (cont'd)	area is characteristic. The rash appears to be photosensitive. Vascular changes and oral lesions may occur, and polyserositis is also present. Renal involvement is very common in childhood SLE.
Juvenile rheumatoid arthritis: Polyarticular	In juvenile rheumatoid arthritis of the polyarticular type, there is multiple joint involvement; frequently, the small joints of the hand are involved. There are pain, tenderness, fusiform swelling, and morning stiffness. Systemic symptoms are uncommon. The temporomandibular joint may be involved, and micrognathia may occur.
Juvenile rheumatoid arthritis: Pauciarticular	Few joints are involved in juvenile rheumatoid arthritis of the pauciarticular type. The symptoms usually occur in the larger joints, such as the knees and elbows. The hips are usually spared. Iridocyclitis occurs and may be the only presenting symptom.
Juvenile rheumatoid arthritis: Systemic	The common symptoms of systemic juvenile rheumatoid arthritis are fever, rash, hepatosplenomegaly, polyarthritis, leukocytosis, serositis, and abdominal pain.
Rheumatic fever	The arthritis of rheumatic fever involves the larger joints and is migratory. The most distal and most proximal joints are usually spared. Swelling, redness, and heat are usually common. Other manifestations are fever, history of sore throat, carditis, subcutaneous nodules, chorea, and erythema marginatum.
Hemophilia	Joint pain may occur when there is bleeding into a joint. There are, typically, swelling and pain with motion. Other signs of a bleeding diathesis may or may not be present.

Rubella	Rubella during childhood is a very mild illness; however, adolescents and adults who contract rubella will commonly have a severe illness characterized by high fever, malaise, myalgia, arthralgia, rash, thrombocytopenia, and petechiae.
Other Causes of Joint Pain	Drugs, gout, typhoid fever, sarcoidosis, syphilis, osteochondritis, mononucleosis, ulcerative colitis, Crohn's disease, and dermatomyositis.

Cause of Joint Pain	Multiple Joints	Small Joints	Large Joints	Arthritis	Effusion Sterile	Fever	Skin Rash	Decreased Complement	Pain with Motion	Lymphadenopathy	Hemarthrosis	Urticaria-Like	GI Symptoms	Renal Symptoms	TM Joint Abnormality	Iridocyclitis	Hepatosplenomegaly	Anemia	Pleuritis and/or Carditis	Subcutaneous Nodules	Leukocytosis	HLA Typing	Drugs
Trauma	1	2	2	0	2	0	0	0	4	0	2	0	0	0	0	0	0	0	0	0	1	0	0
Infection	0	1	3	4	0	4	1	0	4	*	0	0	0	0	0	0	*	0	1	0	4	0	0
Sickle cell disease	4	4	1	0	0	4	0	0	4	0	0	0	1	3	0	0	3	4	0	0	4	0	0
Serum sickness	4	3	3	4	4	3	4	0	3	2	0	4	1	1	0	0	0	0	1	0	2	0	4
Henoch-Schönlein purpura	4	1	4	4	4	4	4	0	4	0	0	3	3	3	0	0	0	0	0	0	3	0	1
SLE	4	4	1	0	4	3	3	4	4	2	0	0	1	4	0	0	1	3	2	1	3	1	1
JRA (polyarticular)	4	4	2	4	4	2	1	0	4	2	0	0	1	1	2	0	2	3	1	2	2	1	1
JRA (pauciarticular)	2	1	4	4	4	2	1	0	4	1	0	0	1	1	1	2	1	2	1	1	2	2-3	0
JRA (systemic)	2	4	2	4	4	4	4	0	4	4	0	0	2	1	0	0	4	3	3	1	3	0	0
Rheumatic fever	4	1	4	3	0	3	1	0	4	1	0	0	2	0	0	0	0	0	4	2	3	0	0
Hemophilia	0	1	4	*	4	0	0	0	4	0	4	0	0	1	0	0	0	*	0	0	0	0	0
Rubella	4	4	4	4	4	2	4	0	4	4	0	0	0	0	0	0	1	0	0	0	0	0	0

Lethargy

Lethargy is described as fatigue, excessive sleepiness, or a decrease in activity.

Important aspects of the history are: Normal patterns: What are the child's normal activity and sleep patterns? Illness: Has the child been ill prior to the onset of the lethargy? Does the child have a fever? Psychological: Is the child doing well in school? Has something occurred in school, with teachers or friends, that may have upset the child? Is there a test in school or homework that was not completed?

The physical examination should focus on signs of infection, signs of central nervous system involvement, and a psychosocial evaluation. In the absence of positive physical findings, psychological evaluation should be pursued in depth.

Fever	Fever from any cause can result in lethargy. Prostration, diaphoresis, and flushing occur with high fevers; myalgia may also be present. Central nervous system infection and sepsis can result in lethargy without significant fever. (Hypothermia may occur with overwhelmingly systemic infections.)
Psychosocial	Depressive states may result in lethargy. Lassitude, drowsiness, fatigue, weakness, and increased sleeping may all be symptoms of psychological stress.
Anemia	Lethargy usually only occurs when the anemia is relatively acute. Adaptation to low hemoglobin usually occurs with chronic anemia. There may be no symptoms, or there may be easy fatigability, drowsiness, pallor, and orthostatic hypotension.

Sepsis/Meningitis	Lethargy may be a symptom of severe systemic infection. Other symptoms that may occur are prostration, meningismus, fever or hypothermia, positive Kernig and Brudzinski signs, convulsions, tachypnea and tachycardia, poor feeding, irritability, vomiting, and diarrhea.
Postictal States	Seizures are frequently followed by a period of lethargy or somnolence.
Infectious Mononucleosis	Malaise, weakness, low grade fever, generalized lymphadenopathy, pharyngitis, periorbital edema, and splenomegaly are signs and symptoms associated with infectious mononucleosis.
Other Causes of Lethargy	Lack of sleep, obesity, puberty, hypoglycemia, drugs, pregnancy, Addison's disease, trauma, and low-grade infection.

Cause of Lethargy

Cause of Lethargy	Tachycardia	Tachypnea	Somnolence or Lassitude	Weakness	Low Hemoglobin	Pallor	Kernig's Sign	Brudzinski's Sign	Vomiting	Diarrhea	Poor Appetite	Seizures	Lymphadenopathy	Splenomegaly
Fever	4	2	2	0	0	0	0	0	0	0	2	0	0	0
Psychological	0	0	4	4	0	0	0	0	0	0	2	0	0	0
Anemia (acute)	3	1	1	2	4	4	0	0	0	0	1	0	*	*
Leukemia	2	1	0	0	3	3	0	0	0	0	1	0	2	2
Meningitis	3	1	2	0	1	0	4	4	3	3	4	1	0	0
Postictal states	0	0	3	4	0	0	0	0	0	0	4	4	0	0
Infectious mononucleosis	0	0	4	2	0	0	0	0	0	0	0	0	4	4
Drug ingestion	0–4	0–4	1	2	0	0	0	0	0	0	2	0	0	0
Head trauma	0–4	0–4	3	0	0	2	0	0	3	0	2	0–4	0	0
Hypoglycemia	3	3	3	2	0	0	0	0	2	0	0	2	0	0

Limp

Gait abnormalities are not uncommon in childhood. An atalgic gait (limp) is characterized by a short steppage phase on the affected extremity. Pain and/or weakness may be present. The diagnosis is generally straightforward and readily apparent from a thorough history and physical examination. The history and clinical examination should be guided by a preconceived hypothesis set. Careful attention should be paid to the onset of the limp, the presence of preceding trauma, and associated signs and symptoms. The limb should be carefully palpated with close attention to the hip, knee, ankle, and plantar aspect of the foot.

Trauma	Trauma is the most common cause of limp in childhood. It may take the form of contusion, sprain, dislocation, or fracture. The history may or may not reveal the traumatic episode. Stress fractures are rare, but do occur, in childhood. The injury may involve any portion of the leg or foot. Physical examination should focus on the foot, lower leg, upper leg, hip, knee, ankle, and toes. Pain and tenderness are usually present. Limitation of motion may occur. Discoloration may be present along with swelling of the involved portion of the extremity. Because of the loose attachment of the periosteum to bone in children, subperiosteal hematoma formation may occur (even with minor trauma). Early radiographs are usually negative, showing calcification only several weeks later.
Foreign Body	Foreign bodies in the foot are not an uncommon cause of limp in children. The history may or may not be positive for the event. The

118

Foreign Body (cont'd)	onset is usually sudden. The foreign body may be readily recognized on physical examination, but occasionally may be occult. The interior surfaces of the child's shoes should be examined when limp is present, or when there is a complaint of foot pain. Poor repair of shoes, protruding tacks, or retained foreign bodies within the shoes may be the cause of the limp.
Infection *Septic arthritis*	Septic arthritis is usually characterized by the sudden onset of fever. The child is usually systemically ill (especially the younger child). Pain, tenderness, limitation of motion, and splinting of the affected joint may occur. Erythema and swelling may be present. If the hip is involved, limp may be the only presenting finding. Fever may be absent early in the disease. In a child who presents with an acute onset of limp, and the etiology cannot be readily ascertained, septic arthritis must be included in the differential diagnosis.
Osteomyelitis	The clinical manifestations of osteomyelitis vary with the location of the infection and with the age of the child. Any bone may be affected. Frequently, it is difficult to differentiate clinically between osteomyelitis and septic arthritis. The patient may or may not appear systemically ill (the younger the child, the more often there are no systemic signs of toxicity). There may be swelling, fever, limitation of motion of the affected bone, warmth, and redness. Radiographic evidence of bone destruction may not be present early in the course of the disease.

Inflammation *Juvenile rheumatoid arthritis*	Small joints of the hands and feet are usually involved in polyarticular disease. Large joints may also be involved. Bilateral involvement is common. Pauciarticular disease (Type 1) usually involves larger joints, which are more often asymmetric.
Synovitis	Synovitis is an entity of unknown etiology which may affect toddlers and older children. Any joint may be involved, but it often affects the hip, knee, or ankle. There may be a history of preceding upper respiratory tract infection. All the signs of inflammation may be present. It is vitally important to not overlook a suppurative infection in the involved joint.
Collagen-vascular disease	Collagen-vascular diseases (e.g., systemic lupus erythematosus, dermatomyositis) are frequently associated with limb and joint pains. Overt inflammation is not uncommon.
Orthopedic Abnormalities *Congenital hip dislocation*	Congenital hip dislocation is most often discovered in the neonatal period. Ortolani's sign (clicking of the hip when flexed and abducted) may be present or the hip may be unstable and dislocatable with downward pressure when flexed. Radiographs are usually diagnostic. Occasionally, a child with congenital hip dislocation will not be diagnosed in the neonatal period. As the child begins to walk, an atalgic gait is usually present.
Legg-Calvé-Perthes' disease	This disorder usually occurs in children between the ages of 4 and 10 years. It may be difficult to distinguish from synovitis or septic arthritis of the hip. A small percentage of children will present with recurrent or persistent synovitis. The onset is usually gradual with the appearance of a limp. Pain is often referred to

Legg-Clavé-Perthes' disease (cont'd)	the knee or anterior thigh. The affected children tend to be slender and/or small for their chronological age.
Slipped capital femoral epiphysis	This entity is most often seen in adolescent obese males. It usually occurs unilaterally, but may be bilateral. The symptoms may mimic synovitis. Pain is frequently referred to the knee.
Nonspecific Leg Pains	Nonspecific pains in the lower limbs are not uncommon in childhood. The pains may be mild or severe, occasionally waking the child from sleep. They are usually self-limited and no abnormalities can be found clinically. Massage and/or the local application of heat may relieve the discomfort. The etiology is unknown. Restlessness may be present. The most common sites are the anterior thigh, calves, and popliteal region. The pains are described as being deep and not associated with a joint. Bilateral involvement is common. Limp is unusual with growing pains and mobility of the affected limb is normal.
Other Causes of Limp	Traumatic arthritis, tendonitis, Osgood-Schlatter's disease, Freiberg's disease, Kohler's disease, tumors, sickle cell disease, vitamin deficiencies, neurological abnormalities (e.g., polio, herniated interveterbral disk), and vertebral spinal abnormalities.

Nystagmus

Nystagmus is the rapid alternating movements of the eyes; patients are usually not significantly disturbed by the movements. The finding of nystagmus on physical examination may be trivial or may be a symptom of significant underlying disease.

The history should determine whether there are any visual problems, as well as the length of time the nystagmus has been present, any ingestion of drugs, the presence of infection, and the presence of any other associated symptoms. Physical examination should focus on the visual and neurological examinations.

Visual Defects	Nystagmus from a visual defect is termed "searching nystagmus," and may result from poor visual acuity, optic atrophy, or astigmatism.
Optic atrophy	Optic atrophy may be unilateral or bilateral. Physical examination reveals pallor of the disk and loss of visual function.
Astigmatism	Astigmatism is a difference in the refractive effect of the corneal meridians; its other symptoms include headache, fatigue, restlessness, school failure, ocular discomfort, and occasional conjunctival hyperemia.
Labyrinthine Nystagmus	The type and degree of labyrinthine nystagmus vary with the head position. There is usually a rotatory component to the nystagmus. The jerking movements of the eyes appear to be greatest with the eyes at rest. Nausea and dizziness are associated with this form of nystagmus.

Congenital Nystagmus	This form of nystagmus is usually described as pendular. There are irregular jerky eye movements on lateral gaze; the eye movements are bilaterally symmetrical. Fixation and visual acuity are usually poor.
Spasmus Nutans	The nystagmus in spasmus nutans, or nodding spasm, is frequently unilateral; when it is bilateral, one eye is more involved than the other. The most common age at onset is between 4 and 12 months. Intermittent head-nodding occurs in 80% of patients.
Drugs	The nystagmus secondary to drugs (e.g., phenytoin) may be due to side effect, idiosyncratic reaction, or overdose. Rhythmic jerking of the eyes is more marked on lateral gaze (this is true also of nystagmus caused by any cerebellar dysfunction). The slow component of the nystagmus is toward the midline.
Cerebellar Ataxia	Nystagmus may be present but is uncommon. Infantile hypotonia, decreased deep tendon reflexes, intention tremors, ataxia, and mild mental retardation may be present.
Albinism *Autosomal recessive albinism*	Autosomal recessive albinism is marked by fair skin, silky hair, gray or blue iris, poor visual acuity secondary to refractive errors, nystagmus, photophobia, and strabismus. The retina may be devoid of pigment.
Autosomal dominant albinism	Autosomal dominant albinism is marked by partial albinism, localized patches of hypopigmented skin, and hair devoid of pigment.
Sex-linked albinism	Sex-linked albinism is marked by ocular albinism and depigmentation of the retina and iris. Nystagmus, photophobia, and poor visual acuity are present.

| Cerebellar Tumor | Cerebellar tumors cause coarse nystagmus. This is exaggerated and is of greater amplitude when the gaze is toward the side on which the tumor is located. |

Cause of Nystagmus	Acute	Chronic	Visual Defect	Retinal Pallor	Pendular	Dizziness	Nausea	Nystagmus Greatest at Rest	Bilateral	Unilateral	Head Nodding	Ataxia	Nonocular Pigment Changes	Photophobia
Optic atrophy	1	3	4	4	3	0	0	0	2	2	0	0	0	0
Astigmatism	0	3	1–4	0	3	2	3	0	2	2	0	0	0	0
Labyrinthine nystagmus	4	1	0	0	3	4	4	4	2	2	0	0–4	0	0
Congenital	0	4	4	0	3	0	0	4	4	0	3	0	0–3	0–4
Spasmus nutans	0	4	0	0	3	0	0	0	1	3	3	0	0	0
Drugs	4	0	0	0	0–3	0–4	0–4	0	4	0	0	2	2	0
Cerebellar infection	4	0	0	0	0	2	2	0	4	0	0	4	0	0
Albinism	0	4	4	4	3	0	0	3	4	0	0	0	3	4
Tumor	0	4	0–4	1	1	0–4	0–4	0	4	0	0	3	0	0

Otalgia

Children frequently complain of earache. The origin of the pain may be external or internal to the tympanic membrane. The tympanic membrane itself may be involved. Referred pain to the ear may also be present, and etiologies from systems other than the auditory system should be considered.

Hard Wax	Large collections of hard wax may cause discomfort secondary to direct irritation of the external auditory canal. The cerumen can be seen directly.
Otitis Externa	Ear pain may be significant. There is frequently preauricular tenderness, as well as pain with movement of the pinna. There may be periauricular swelling. Exudate may be present.
Otitis Media	The degree of otalgia is variable. Fever is frequently present with suppurative otitis media. The external canal is normal. The tympanic membrane bulges, and there is complete loss of normal tympanic membrane landmarks. Otalgia may also occur with nonsuppurative forms of otitis media (e.g., serous otitis, secretory otitis). There may be tympanic membrane retraction and/or air-fluid levels.
Bullous Myringitis	This is an extremely painful condition. Fever may or may not be present. Serous bullae form on the tympanic membrane and may be easily visualized. The pain is relieved with rupture of the blebs. Occasionally, the bullae are hemorrhagic.

Furuncle/ Carbuncle	These may be very painful and tender. They occur in the skin of the external auditory canal and may be easily visualized.
Foreign Body	Ear pain associated with foul-smelling discharge is suggestive of a foreign body.
Other Causes of Otalgia	Pinna injury, eczema/seborrhea, frostbite, mastoiditis, and referred pain from the teeth, mouth, and pharynx.

Cause of Otalgia	Excessive Cerumen	Preauricular Tenderness	Pain with Movement of Pinna	Periauricular Swelling	Exudate in Canal	Fever	Bulging Drums	Retracted Drums	Loss of Normal Landmarks	Poor Tympanic Membrane Compliance	Bullae	Fluid	Localized Swelling in Canal	Foul-Smelling Discharge
Hard wax	4	0	0	0	0	0	0	0	3	0	0	0	0	0
Otitis externa	0	3	4	2	2	1	0	0	0	0	0	0	0	0
Otitis media	0	0	0	0	0	4	3	0	4	4	1	3	0	0
Bullous myringitis	0	0	0	0	0	2	2	0	0	2	4	2	0	0
Furuncle/carbuncle	0	1	2	0	0	0	0	0	0	0	0	0	4	0
Foreign body	0	0	0	0	2	0	0	0	*	0	0	0	2	4
Trauma to canal	0	2	3	2	1	0	0	0	0	0	0	0	0	0
Secretory otitis	0	0	0	0	0	0	0	3	2	4	0	4	0	0

Photophobia

Photophobia is the "fear of light." The meaning is expanded to signify any situation in which there is an aversion to light (usually a painful or uncomfortable sensation to normal lighting conditions).

Photophobia is, rarely, an isolated syndrome. It is most commonly associated with other local or systemic signs and symptoms. The history should focus on the following: Is there burning, itching, redness, swelling, or pain in the eyes? Has there been a rash? Was the onset acute or has the problem been present for a long time? Are there symptoms of urinary tract infection?

Manifestations of systemic illness, as well as local ocular disease, should be sought.

Conjunctivitis	Conjunctivitis is a common disorder of childhood. There is hyperemia of the palpebral and/or bulbar conjunctivae, with perilimbal sparing. The discharge may vary from simple epiphoria to a purulent discharge. There may be a sensation of a foreign body in the eye. The cornea, pupil, and vision are normal.
Uveitis	This is an uncommon condition characterized by ocular pain and photophobia, epiphoria, circumcorneal hyperemia, and an irregular, meiotic pupil. Vision is poor. The anterior chamber may be cloudy.
Keratitis	Keratitis frequently follows trauma to the cornea or may be the result of infection of the cornea. There are significant eye pain, epiphoria, photophobia, and circumcorneal hyperemia. The cornea may appear cloudy. The pupil is normal.

| Glaucoma | Glaucoma is characterized by photophobia, epiphoria, meiosis, cloudy cornea, poor vision, and elevated ocular tension. |
| Other Causes of Photophobia | Vitamin A deficiency, blepharitis, albinism, mercury intoxication, phlyctenular conjunctivitis, and meningitis. |

Cause of Photophobia	Hyperemia	Perilimbal Pallor	Epiphora	Purulent Discharge	Foreign Body Sensation	Pain	Circumcorneal Flush	Constricted Pupil	Dilated Pupil	Poor Vision	Cloudy Anterior Chamber	Cloudy Cornea	Increased Ocular Tension
Conjunctivitis	4	3	1	3	2	1	0	0	0	0	0	0	0
Uveitis	3	0	4	0	1	4	4	4	0	3	3	0	0
Keratitis	3	0	0	0	1	4	4	0	0	2	0	4	0
Glaucoma	0	0	4	0	0	0	0	4	0	4	0	4	4
Drugs	0	0	0-4	0	0	0	0	0-4	0-4	0	0	0	0-4
Trauma	4	0	0-4	0	4	3	0	0-4	0-4	0-4	0	0	0-4

Proteinuria

Isolated proteinuria is usually considered the presence of >50 mg/dl or > 200 mg/24 hours of protein in an otherwise normal urine specimen. A small amount of protein (albumin) in the urine is not abnormal. Symptomatic children may present with edema, growth failure, and/or hypertension. The presence of blood and/or casts in the urine sample usually signifies a nephritic etiology for the proteinuria. If blood is present in the urine, specific diagnostic protocols should be followed for appropriate evaluation.

Causes of Asymptomatic Proteinuria	Orthostatic, exercise-induced, fever, allergic, and prenephrotic.
Causes of Symptomatic Proteinuria	Primary renal disease, renal dysplasia, chronic pyelonephritis, hydronephrosis, nephrotic syndrome, renal vein thrombosis, diabetes mellitus, collagen-vascular diseases, hemoglobinuria, renal tubular disorders, Wilson's disease, and Fanconi's syndrome.

Ptosis

Ptosis means the drooping of one or both eyelids. It is also termed blepharoptosis. This symptom is unusual in childhood and almost always indicates a pathological condition. True ptosis must be differentiated from pseudoptosis, a condition in which the eyelid(s) only appears to droop. Attention must be paid to the history, especially the age at onset of the ptosis, the acuteness of onset, and the presence of a family history.

Pseudoptosis	This may occur in the newborn when there is asymmetrical opening of the eyes. Mild edema of one or both lids may cause pseudoptosis.
Congenital Ptosis	This is an autosomal dominant trait characterized by defective or absent development of the levator muscle. It may be unilateral or bilateral. Children may use their frontalis muscle or tilt their head backward to maintain vision. Ipsilateral superior rectus palsy, epicanthal folds, and strabismus may be associated findings. It may be associated with Turner's syndrome or Fabry's disease.
Marcus Gunn Phenomenon	Marcus Gunn phenomenon is termed "jaw-winking." There is an anomalous connection between the external pterygoid muscle and the levator muscle. Ptosis is present. Movement of the jaw to one side or protrusion of the jaw causes elevation of the contralateral eyelid.
Myasthenia Gravis	Ptosis is often present in myasthenia gravis and is often the presenting finding. Generalized weakness occurs and usually increases with exercise. There is improvement of strength

Myasthenia Gravis (cont'd)	and resolution of the ptosis after the administration of Tensilon®.
Other Causes of Ptosis	CNS tumors, trauma, poisoning, oculomotor paralysis, Parinaud's syndrome, Möbius syndrome, Horner's syndrome, postencephalitis, Smith-Lemli-Opitz syndrome, Zellweger's syndrome, myotonic dystrophy, and botulism.

Puberty, Delayed (Female)

PRIMARY AMENORREA

Primary amenorrhea is described as the absence of menarche by age 16 years. Delayed puberty is the delay in appearance of secondary sexual characteristics. The onset of pubescent changes in girls generally occurs between 8 and 13 years of age.

The time of puberty and menarche of the patient's mother and female siblings must be obtained in the history.

The normal order of appearance of secondary sexual characteristics is as follows: (1) increased pelvic width, (2) breast development, (3) pubic hair, (4) axillary hair, (5) change from alkaline to acid vaginal secretion, and (6) menarche generally occurs two years after breast development begins.

Etiologies of Primary Amenorrhea	Constitutional, malnutrition, chronic illness, Turner syndrome, pituitary dwarfism, gonadotropin deficiency, absent vagina or uterus, ovarian cyst or tumor, adrenal hyperplasia, and testicular feminization.

SECONDARY AMENORRHEA

Secondary amenorrhea is defined as any cessation of menses after menarche has occurred. There are few etiologies.

Historical evaluation should include questions relating to: (1) the age of menarche, (2) the explanation of normal cycles, (3) the duration of menses, (4) the presence or absence of dysmenorrhea, (5) breast enlargement, (6) vomiting, fatigue, or abdominal pain, (7) sexual activity and the use of contraception, (8) eating problems, and (9) associated illnesses.

Pregnancy	Presumptive evidence of pregnancy includes secondary amenorrhea, breast swelling, hyperpigmentation of the areola, enlargement of the uterus, and fatigue. Definitive diagnosis is made by auscultation of the fetal heart beat, palpation of fetal parts, or visualization of the fetal skeleton on X-ray film or sonography.
Anovulatory Cycles	Amenorrhea secondary to anovulatory cycles occurs near menarche. Menses are extremely irregular but usually painless.
Other Causes of Secondary Amenorrhea	Chronic illness, emotional stress, and anorexia nervosa.

Puberty, Delayed (Male)

Delayed puberty in males is the failure of secondary sex characteristics to appear by the age of 16 years.

The family history should be investigated for ages at onset of puberty in the father and other male siblings. The normal range of onset of puberty in boys is 10 to 14 years. There is some variability in their appearance, but, generally, the sexual changes are as follows: (1) increase in size of the scrotum and testes, (2) increase in size of the penis, (3) occasional unilateral breast swelling, (4) pubic hair, (5) axillary hair, and (6) facial hair.

The physical examination must include a complete examination of the genitalia. The testes should be palpated and evaluated for size, consistency, and the presence of masses. If the testes are not palpable in the scrotal sac, the inguinal canals must be thoroughly palpated.

Laboratory evaluations that may be of aid in establishing a diagnosis are chromosome studies, urinary 17-ketosteroids and gonadotropins, skull X-ray series, and pituitary function testing.

Etiologies of Delayed Puberty in Males	Constitutional, malnutrition, chronic illness (e.g., sickle cell anemia), tuberculosis, diabetes mellitus, rheumatic fever, Crohn's disease, ulcerative colitis, pituitary etiologies, cryptorchidism, Klinefelter's syndrome, and pseudohermaphroditism.

Purpura

The term purpura is derived from the name *Purpura lapillus*, a fish from which purple dye was made. The term was used by the Greeks and Romans to describe the color purple; it has evolved to take on a more limited meaning.

Purpura is used to designate any hemorrhage into the skin. These may take the form of small pinpoint hemorrhages (petechiae) or larger areas of hemorrhage (ecchymosis). There are two common classifications of purpura: Purpura with low platelet counts (thrombocytopenic purpura) and purpura with normal platelet counts (nonthrombocytopenic purpura).

The age of the patient may yield clues to the etiology. An accurate history regarding allergies, drugs, and prior illnesses is necessary. The family history may point to hereditary or congenital etiologies. Search for signs of trauma or abuse.

Etiologies of Purpura in the Newborn Period	Birth trauma, maternal thrombocytopenia, drugs (maternal quinine and chlorothiazide), hemolytic disease of the newborn, sepsis, congenital syphilis, large hemangiomas, congenital leukemia, toxoplasmosis, cytomegalovirus infection, congenital herpesvirus infection, congenital rubella, galactosemia, and thrombocytopenia with absent radius (TAR) syndrome.
Thrombocytopenic Purpura *Idiopathic (ITP)*	Greatest frequency is between the ages of 2 and 8 years. There are two forms: acute and chronic (with remissions). The acute form has a sudden onset of thrombocytopenia and purpura. It frequently follows a viral infection. In both forms a common presenting complaint is

Thrombocyto-penic Purpura *Idiopathic (ITP)* (cont'd)	easy bruising. There may be diffuse petechiae and ecchymosis. Sites of bleeding frequently seen at the onset of the condition are the nasal, gingival, and oral mucosa, gastrointestinal tract, urinary tract, and vagina. Petechiae and ecchymosis are commonly found in the gluteal region and over bony prominences. The spleen is usually not palpable. The platelet count is usually below 50,000/mm³. Bleeding time is prolonged; clot retraction is poor, prothrombin time is normal. Bone marrow examination reveals normal or increased megakaryocytes with reduced platelet formation.
Congenital	This condition occurs in infants born of mothers with thrombocytopenia. An isoimmune etiology (similar to Rh incompatibility) has been identified. Petechiae are common. Other areas of bleeding are uncommon. The platelet counts in these infants usually return to normal within 2 to 3 weeks.
Infections	Rubella, syphilis, toxoplasmosis, cytomegalovirus, bacterial sepsis, subacute bacterial endocarditis, typhoid, rubeola, varicella, scarlet fever, variola, and Rocky Mountain spotted fever are all infectious causes of purpura.
Drugs and chemicals	Thyroid suppressing agents, quinine, certain thiazides, mesantoin, arsenic, chloramphenicol, and cancer chemotherapeutic agents.
Aplastic anemia	Associated with the thrombocytopenia are severe anemia and granulocytopenia, with an extremely low or absent reticulocyte count.
Thrombotic (TTP)	This is a fulminating purpuric disease characterized by acute onset, fever, severe hemolytic anemia, and neurological signs (which may be focal or generalized). The brain, kidney, heart, and spleen are involved.

Wiskott-Aldrich syndrome	Recurrent infection, eczema, and thrombocytopenic purpura form the classic triad in Wiskott-Aldrich syndrome. Recurrent otitis media, bloody diarrhea, epistaxis, anemia, pansinusitis, bronchopneumonia, skin infection, and meningitis may occur. Hepatosplenomegaly may be present.
Hemolytic-uremic syndrome	The characteristic age at which this condition occurs is from infancy to 7 years. The classic features are hemolytic anemia, thrombocytopenia, and acute renal failure. Onset of the syndrome is almost always preceded by abdominal pain and bloody diarrhea (by 3 days to 6 weeks in one series) that may be mistaken for gastroenteritis, appendicitis, ulcerative colitis, or Crohn's disease. Hypertension, oliguria, and hematuria may be present. Central nervous system manifestations (irritability, lethargy, convulsions, and coma) may occur. Fibrinogen, prothrombin, and factors V and VII are commonly decreased.
Kasabach-Merritt syndrome	This condition is marked by petechiae and ecchymosis, as well as other bleeding tendencies secondary to sequestration of platelets and other coagulation factors in large hemangiomas. Disseminated intravascular coagulation may account for the bleeding.
Other causes of thrombocytopenic purpura	X-ray exposure, neoplasms, marrow fibrosis, autoimmune hemolytic anemia, pernicious anemia of childhood, hypersplenism, Gaucher's disease, systemic lupus erythematosus (SLE), Felty's syndrome, Banti's syndrome, infectious mononucleosis, and blood transfusion.

Nonthrombocytopenic Purpura *Trauma (child abuse)*	The presence of a pattern of multiple ecchymotic areas (especially in various stages of resolution) with normal coagulation studies should alert the examiner to the possibility of child abuse.
Henoch-Schönlein purpura	Henoch-Schönlein purpura, or "anaphylactoid purpura," most commonly affects children between the ages of 2 and 15 years. At onset there may be fever, cephalgia, and abdominal pain. Urticarial lesions appear, which may develop petechiae in the erythematous region of the wheal/flare reaction. The lesions progress to ecchymosis. Skin manifestations are most common over the buttocks, low back, and posterior aspect of the legs and arms. Colicky abdominal pain is striking, and the clinical picture may resemble that in intussusception. There may be transient swelling of the knees and ankles, or frank arthritic symptoms may be present. Soft tissue edema may be present. Glomerulonephritis may occur (50% of patients). There may be hematuria and proteinuria. The platelet count and coagulation studies are normal.
Meningococcemia	Children with meningococcemia are acutely ill, with purpura appearing 24 to 48 hours after onset of illness. Meningeal signs may be present. Petechiae, ecchymosis, or purpura in the presence of meningeal signs signifies meningococcus infection until proven otherwise.
Hereditary hemorrhagic telangiectasia	Hereditary hemorrhagic telangiectasia, or Rendu-Weber-Osler disease, is marked by diffuse telangiectasias that tend to bleed spontaneously or after minor trauma. A frequent presentation is recurrent epistaxis.

Von Willebrand disease	Also called pseudohemophilia. There is a prolonged bleeding time; the clotting time and platelet counts are normal. There may be abnormal platelet adhesiveness. A capillary defect is described. Excessive spontaneous epistaxis and bleeding from the gingivae are common presenting symptoms. Bruising occurs easily. There is an associated factor VIII deficiency.
Ehler-Danlos syndrome	Clinical features of this syndrome are hyperextensibility of joints, hyperelasticity of skin, extreme friability of skin and blood vessels, and subcutaneous nodules. Rupture of arteries and aneurysmal lesions may occur. Bleeding and coagulation studies are usually normal.
Purpura fulminans	This is a severe disease characterized by the acute onset of shock, fever, anemia, and progressive purpura; it frequently follows an infectious disease, with scarlet fever being the most common of the preceding conditions.

Retinal Hemorrhage

Retinal hemorrhage is an uncommon finding in children. If present, it usually signifies significant underlying pathology.

Patients with retinal hemorrhage usually present with symptoms other than visual problems, and the hemorrhage is found incidentally on physical examination. Historical questioning should be guided by the presenting signs and symptoms of the underlying disease process.

Hypertension	In patients with hypertension, retinal hemorrhage usually signifies longstanding or severe malignant hypertension. The patient may be asymptomatic or headache, convulsion, hematuria, or epistaxis may occur.
Diabetes Mellitus	Diabetic retinopathy is uncommon in the pediatric population. When it does occur, it is severe, and blindness rapidly ensues. Other signs of complications of diabetes are usually present, such as renal disease and frequent, resistant infection.
Blood Dyscrasias	The initial sign of a bleeding disorder may be retinal hemorrhage. Retinal hemorrhage may also be found in patients with hemoglobin SS (classic sickle cell anemia) or SC [a disease in which there is a combination of hemoglobin S (sickle hemoglobin) and hemoglobin C. The manifestations of hemoglobin SC disease are similar to those of sickle cell anemia but may be more mild]. Hematuria and retinal hemorrhage may occur in both SS and SC disease.
Trauma/ Child Abuse	Retinal hemorrhage may occur secondary to ocular trauma. If no organic etiology can be

Trauma/Child Abuse (cont'd)	found and the history is inconsistent with the physical findings, child abuse should be suspected.
Other Causes of Retinal Hemorrhage	Retrobulbar neuritis, subdural hemotoma, pertussis, telangiectasia, and ocular tumor.

Cause of Retinal Hemorrhage	Headaches	Epistaxis	Loss of Vision	Purpura	Anemia	Decreased Clotting Factors	History of Trauma	Pain
Hypertension	2	1	1	0	0	0	0	0
Diabetes mellitus	0	0	1	0	0	0	0	0
Blood dyscrasia	0	3	1	4	3	2	0	0
Trauma	0	1	1	0	0	0	4	0
Retrobulbar neuritis	1	0	3	0	0	0	0	4
Tumor	3	0	3	0	0	0	0	0
Coagulopathies	1	3	1	3	3	4	0	0

Seizures

Seizures are symptoms of central nervous system irritation. Their manifestations depend on the location of the seizure focus in the brain, as well as on the seizure progression or spread. The symptomatology may vary from a generalized tonic–clonic major motor seizure, to absence spells, flashes of light, or recurrent stomach pain. Seizures are most often intermittent and paroxysmal. They may or may not be preceded by an aura or followed by a postictal state.

The etiologies of seizures are as varied as their manifestations. The majority of underlying causes are simply listed in the differential diagnosis, since most are self-explanatory. Only the differentiation between simple febrile convulsions, febrile seizures, and afebrile seizures is discussed more fully. The remaining etiologies appear according to the age group in which they are most likely to occur.

Simple Febrile Convulsions	Simple febrile convulsions occur in children from 6 months to 6 years of age. These seizures are benign and self-limited; the child is previously normal, and there is no evidence of neurological deficit. The seizure is usually generalized and may occur as early as 2 hours after the onset of the fever. The fever may be from any cause (e.g., otitis media, roseola infantum); however, central nervous system infection is, by definition, not present. The electroencephalogram (EEG) is usually normal. In the case of any febrile convulsion, meningitis or other central nervous system infection must be ruled out.

Seizures with Fever	Breakthrough seizures may occur with fever in any seizure disorder. (Seizure disorder is usually an underlying condition.) These children may have afebrile seizures as well. Seizures can occur at any age notwithstanding fever. This type of seizure may occur in previously abnormal children. Neurological deficits may be present. The seizures may be focal or generalized. The EEG may be abnormal. In general, fever decreases the seizure threshold in those children and adolescents with afebrile seizures. Again, central nervous system infection must be ruled out.
Afebrile Seizures	Afebrile seizures occur in the absence of fever. They may take any form, from major motor seizures to epileptic equivalents. They are almost always accompanied by altered levels of consciousness.
Etiologies of Seizures in the Neonatal Period	Hypoxia, sepsis, meningitis, encephalitis, hypoglycemia, hypocalcemia, hypomagnesemia, electrolyte imbalance, metabolic defects, pyridoxine deficiency, narcotic withdrawal, maternal drug use, central nervous system deformity, cerebral hemorrhage, neonatal tetanus, and infantile spasm.
Etiologies of Seizures in Infancy and Early Childhood	Simple febrile convulsions, epilepsy, meningitis, encephalitis, brain abcess, sepsis, intracranial tumors, intracranial hemorrhage, trauma, infantile spasm, metabolic abnormalities, diabetes, hypoglycemia, electrolyte imbalance, uremia, hemolytic-uremic syndrome, Reye's syndrome, and drugs (alcohol, lead, and poisons).

| Etiologies of Seizures in Later Childhood and Adolescence | Meningitis, encephalitis, brain abscess, tumor, epilepsy, drugs/poisons, psychological problems, trauma, hypoglycemia, diabetes, hypertension, hemolytic-uremic syndrome, hyperventilation, dehydration, uremia, and Reye's syndrome. |

Cause of Seizures	Age of Patient	Focal	Generalized	Fever	Meningismus	Decreased CSF Glucose	CSF Pleocytosis	Focal EEG Changes	Vomiting	Aura	Family History	Prolonged	Amnesia for Event
Simple febrile convulsion	4	0	4	4	0	0	0	0	0	0	4	0	4
Epilepsy	0	1	3	0	0	0	0	1	0	2	2	0	2
Infection	0	1	3	4	4	4	4	0	2	0	0	2	2
Trauma	0	1	3	0	0	0	0	4	3	0	0	2	4
Tumor	0	1	3	0	0	0	0	4	1	0	0	0	2
Drug ingestion/intoxication	0	0	4	0	0	0	0	0	1	1	0	3	0

Sexual Precocity (Male and Female)

Sexual precocity is the premature development of secondary sex characteristics. This may occur during infancy, denoting possibly significant underlying disease, or in late childhood, which may be normal—constitutional, early isosexual development.

Precocious sexual development may be isosexual or heterosexual. It may take the form of masculinization or feminization.

It is important to determine the age at which the parents experienced puberty, the parents' stature, and the development of siblings.

Female Constitutional	Early thelarche and pubarche may occur normally in a child when sexual maturation occurred at an early age in the parents.
McCune–Albright's syndrome	In McCune–Albright's syndrome (polyostotic fibrous dysplasia), there are fibrous dysplasia of bone, patchy cutaneous pigmentation, and sexual precocity. Cushing's syndrome and hyperthyroidism may also be present.
Adrenogenital syndrome	Salt-losing adrenogenital syndrome: Female children with this condition have enlarged clitorises. There are weight loss, dehydration, vomiting, diarrhea, anorexia, and cardiac disturbance.
Other causes of female sexual precocity	Adrenal tumor, ovarian granulous cell tumor, and teratoma.

Male *Constitutional*	As in the female, early isosexual development may be genetically determined by the age at which the parents reached sexual maturity.
Adrenal hyperplasia	In the salt-sparing form of the adrenogenital syndrome, there is premature isosexual development of the male (and pseudohermaphroiditism in the female). In the salt-losing form of the syndrome, the genitalia of the male may appear normal. Vomiting, weight loss, dehydration, diarrhea, anorexia, and cardiac disturbances may be present.
Adrenal tumor	Premature isosexual development may occur. The tumor may be palpated or may be suspected by kidney displacement, as seen during IVP.
Other causes of male sexual precocity	Hydrocephalus and postencephalitis.

Cause of Sexual Precocity	Other Family Members	Bone Abnormalities	Hyperthyroid	Cushing's Syndrome	Vomiting	Diarrhea	Electrolyte Abnormalities	CNS Abnormalities
Constitutional	1	*	0	0	0	0	0	0
McCune-Albright's disease	0	4	1	1	0	0	0	0
Adrenogenital syndrome	0	*	0	0	4	4	4	0
Tumor	0	*	0	2	0	0	0	1
Postencephalitis	0	*	0	0	0	0	0	4
Hydrocephalus	0	*	0	0	0	0	0	4

Stiff Neck

The child with a stiff neck will frequently alarm parents, who will seek early medical advice. The time of onset, prior or recent illness, presence of fever, and ingestion of medications should all be investigated in the history. In the physical examination, a search should be made for the presence of adenopathy, pharyngitis, otitis media, joint manifestations, and signs of systemic infection.

Meningitis Encephalitis	When a child presents with a stiff neck, central nervous system (CNS) infections should be considered first. A child with CNS infection will look sick and resist movement. There is involuntary splinting of the neck to resist traction on the meninges. Fever, irritability, lethargy, poor feeding, vomiting, diarrhea, acidosis, focal neurological signs, seizures, and coma are all symptoms that may be present in a child with sepsis or meningitis. The younger the child, the less specific the symptoms. Signs of meningeal irritation may be conspicuously absent. A high index of suspicion is necessary when evaluating children less than 2 years of age for meningitis.
Cervical Lymphadenitis (Including Pharyngitis)	Viral or bacterial pharyngitis, as well as primary or secondary cervical lymphadenitis, may result in splinting of the neck. Pain is usually unilateral, and there will be full range of motion to the side opposite the involvement. The lymph nodes may be palpable and tender.
Neck Trauma	Trauma to the neck, such as a blow or "whiplash" can cause contusion to the muscles and ligaments. There are splinting of the neck sec-

Neck Trauma (cont'd)	ondary to pain and/or traumatic inflammation of the muscle/connective tissue structures.
Acute Torticollis	There is acute spasm of the sternocleido-mastoid muscle. The head is flexed laterally toward the side of the spasm, and the chin is rotated away from the side of the spasm. The etiology may be viral. Myositis may be present.
Other Causes of Stiff Neck	Intracranial hemorrhage, tumor or abscess, drugs, postlumbar puncture, retropharyngeal abscess, sternocleidomastoid hematoma, and vertebral anomaly.

Cause of Stiff Neck

Cause of Stiff Neck	Prior Illness	Fever	Medications	Cephalgia	Sore Throat	Otalgia	History of Trauma	Unilateral (Pain)	Bilateral (Pain)	Adenopathy	Focal Neurological Signs
Meningitis/encephalitis	3	4	0	4	0	0	0	0	4	0	1
Cervical lymphadenopathy	3	1	0	2	3	2	0	3	2	4	0
Trauma	0	0	0	2	0	0	4	3	0	0	1
Torticollis	0	0	1	0	0	0	0	4	0	0	0
Intracranial space-occupying lesion	0	0	0	4	0	0	0	0	0–4	0	2
Otitis media	3	3	0	3	1	4	0	2	2	2	0
Retropharyngeal abscess	4	4	1	0	4	1	0	1–4	0	3	0

Stool Color

The color and characteristics of the stool can give much information regarding the diet and the presence or absence of an active disease process. It is important to determine the exact color of the stool, its consistency, any unusual odor, and the frequency of defecation.

Gross examination of the stool may reveal blood, undigested food products, foreign bodies, mucus, or fat. Simple tests for stool pH, the presence of reducing substances, and the presence of blood or fat can be performed rapidly and inexpensively.

Red	A red color to the stool may indicate gross blood; however, ampicillin, as well as red gelatin products, can impart a pinkish color to the stool.
White/Clay-Colored	White stools may indicate a previous barium meal or ingestion of aluminum hydroxide preparations. Clay-colored stools are usually indicative of biliary obstruction or malabsorption.
Black	Black stools may indicate increased iron in the diet, blood, or charcoal, or may be suggestive of pica.
Green/ Greenish Gold	Gastroenteritis in young children frequently presents with green mucoid stools. A greenish-gold colored stool is normal in the fully breast-fed baby. Greenish stools may be indicative of hypermobility of the gut.
Yellow	A normal formula stool is described as mushy, yellow, and seedy.

Stridor

Stridor is described as harsh, "crowing," or noisy respiration. It may be high or low pitched. It may be inspiratory, expiratory, or both. The stridor may be acute in onset or may be present from birth. Stridor may be associated with hoarseness.

It is important to determine whether the child was ill prior to the onset of the stridor. Was the onset acute or had it been present for a long time? Was the patient eating at the time of onset? Is the throat sore? Has there been trauma to the head or neck? Does the patient frequently put foreign objects into his or her mouth? Is there a history of heart disease?

Care should be taken in examining the pharynx in children with stridor, since with certain etiologies, laryngospasm and complete airway obstruction may result after slight stimulation. The physical examination should focus on the following: Character of the stridor: What is the tonal quality of the stridor? The quality may yield clues to the location of the pathology (supraglottic, glottic, or subglottic). Is it inspiratory, expiratory, or both? Is it constant or intermittent? Mouth and pharynx: Is the throat red? Is exudate present? Can the epiglottis be seen? Neck: Is the trachea in the midline? Are there any extrinsic masses? Is there evidence of trauma? Severity of airway obstruction: Is there respiratory distress or cyanosis?

The etiologies will be separated into "acute" and "chronic."

Stridor of Acute Onset *Foreign body*	The most common age group is that from 6 months to 2 years. Foreign bodies lodged in the supraglottic, glottic, or subglottic region, or the trachea, can cause stridor. The history

157

Stridor of **Acute Onset** 　*Foreign body* 　(cont'd)	may be positive for the ingestion. The stridor may be inspiratory, expiratory, or both. The degree of respiratory distress is variable. Cough is usually present. A pretracheal "slap" may be palpated, as well as an audible "thud." Aphonia may be present. Wheezing and cyanosis may occur.
Epiglottitis	The onset of acute epiglottitis is rapid. The initial symptoms depend upon the age of the patient. The older patient may initially complain of sore throat and difficulty in swallowing. Respiratory distress rapidly follows. The stridor may be inspiratory, expiratory, or both. The patient may drool excessively and frequently look very anxious. Examination of the pharynx may reveal a cherry-red epiglottis. Lateral radiographs of the neck may demonstrate the edematous epiglottis (thumb sign).
Laryngo- *tracheo-* *bronchitis* *(LTB)*	Symptoms of coryza followed by a brassy cough and inspiratory stridor may indicate LTB. Fever is usually low grade. The onset is most frequently insidious.
Trauma	Any trauma to the larynx or trachea may cause stridor. There may be deformity of the larynx or paralysis of the vocal cords. The degree of stridor is variable, as is the degree of respiratory distress.
Other causes *of stridor of* *acute onset*	Laryngospasm, diphtheria, and retropharyngeal abscess.
Stridor of **Chronic Onset** 　*Laryngo-* 　*malaria/* 　*tracheo-* 　*malaria*	The stridor is inspiratory. There is noisy, "crowing" breathing. There may be hoarseness, aphonia, dyspnea, or varying degrees of respiratory distress. The stridor appears after the first few days of life, or may be present at birth.

Vocal cord paralysis	There may be unilateral or bilateral paralysis. If unilateral, stridor and respiratory distress are usually minimal, and hoarseness may be the only symptom. If paralysis is bilateral, stridor and distress may be severe. There may be a history of trauma.
Other causes of stridor of chronic onset	Laryngeal webs, congenital subglottic stenosis, laryngeal cyst, micrognathia, thyroglossal duct cyst, vascular ring, missed foreign body, and tumors.

Cause of Stridor	Acute Onset	Slow Onset	Chronic	Sore Throat	History of Foreign Object	Inspiratory	Expiratory	Inspiratory/Expiratory	Fever	Wheezing	Drooling	Cyanosis	Respiratory Distress	Aphonia	Cough	Dysphagia
Spasmotic croup	4	0	0	0	0	4	0	0	0	0	0	0	0	1	4	0
Foreign body	4	0	0	3	4	2	2	2	0	2	0	1	2	2	3	1
LTB	2	2	0	1	0	4	0	0	3	0	0	*	*	0–2	4	0
Epiglottitis	4	0	0	3	0	4	0	0	4	0	4	*	3	1	1	3
Trauma	4	0	1	0	0	1–4	1–4	1–4	0	0	0	*	1–4	1–4	3	0
Laryngomalacia	4	0	4	0	0	4	1	1	0	0	0	0	0	0	0	0
Vocal cord paralysis	2	2	4	0	0	1–4	1–4	1–4	0	0	0	*	1–4	4	1	0
Diphtheria	0	0	0	4	0	4	1	1	3	0	1	*	*	0	3	3
Tumors	0	4	3	0–3	0	0–4	0–4	0–4	0–2	1	0	0	0	0	0–2	1–2

Vaginal Bleeding

Vaginal bleeding in infants (and in girls who have not reached menarche) usually provokes the parents to seek early medical advice. Bleeding after menarche does not cause the same concern. Therefore, in establishing a differential diagnosis, the patient's age is of great importance.

The history should include questions pursuant to the following: Has there been any trauma? Has the patient reached menarche? Have there been any sexual contacts? Does the patient masturbate? Could the patient have inserted a foreign object into the vagina? Is there associated pain? Are there symptoms referable to the urinary tract? Is there a history of bleeding disorders? Is the patient taking any medications or drugs? Has there been a recent gynecological examination?

Physical examination should include a complete inspection of the perineum, a vaginal examination, and a rectal examination.

Menarche	The onset of menses should be considered in the differential diagnosis of vaginal bleeding. Menarche usually occurs approximately two years after the onset of thelarche.
Normal Menstruation	Vaginal bleeding may be part of normal menstruation.
Dysfunctional Uterine Bleeding	Dysfunctional uterine bleeding may take the form of menorrhagia, metorrhagia, or irregularity of menses.
Estrogen Withdrawal	In the mature female on oral contraceptives, withdrawal of estrogen will cause the endometrium to slough. In newborn females, withdrawal of maternal estrogen, caused by placental separation, may cause vaginal bleeding.

Breakthrough Bleeding	This occurs in women taking estrogen-containing oral contraceptives. When the contraceptive does not contain enough estrogen to support the endometrium, sloughing will occur.
Trauma/Abuse	Trauma and child abuse should be considered in all premenarchal females with vaginal bleeding, and perineal irritation or injury.
Foreign Body	Bleeding may occur if a foreign body is inserted into the vagina. There may be a profuse, foul-smelling discharge. The foreign body may be palpated on rectal examination.
Implantation Sign	Implantation of the embryo into the endometrium is frequently associated with a small amount of vaginal bleeding. Other presumptive signs of pregnancy may be present.
Other Causes of Vaginal Bleeding	Tumor and blood dyscrasias.

Cause of Vaginal Bleeding	Premenarchal	Menarche	Postmenarchal	History of Trauma	Sexual Contact	Dysuria	Hematuria	Frequency	Urgency	Medication History	Pain	Bruises Easily	Excessive or Prolonged Bleeding	Foul-Smelling Discharge	Abdominal and/or Adnexal Tenderness
Menarche	0	4	0	0	0	0	0	0	0	0	0–4	0	0	0	1
Menstruation	0	*	4	0	0	0	0	0	0	0	0–4	0	0	0	1
Dysfunctional uterine bleeding	4	1	3	0	0	0	0	0	0	0–4	0	0	4	0	0
Estrogen withdrawal	4	4	4	0	0	0	0	0	0	4	0	0	4	0	0
Trauma	0–4	0–4	0–4	4	*	0	0	0	0	0	4	0	3	0	1
Foreign body	0–4	0–4	0–4	1	0	2	2	2	2	0	3	0	3	3	3
Pregnancy (ectopic)	0	1	3	0	4	0	0	0	0	0	3	0	4	0	4
Pregnancy (spontaneous abortion)	0	1	3	0	4	0	0	0	0	1	3	0	3	1	3
Blood dyscrasias	0	1	3	0	0	0	1	0	0	0	0	4	4	0	0

Vertigo

Vertigo is the subjective sensation of dizziness. It may be a symptom indicating significant underlying pathology. Before psychological factors are considered, organic pathology must be ruled out.

Specific lines of historical questioning are: Time of onset: When does the dizziness occur? Is there an awareness (aura) that an episode of vertigo may occur? Do the episodes occur before or after meals? Does eating relieve the dizziness? Prior illnesses: Have there been any illnesses prior to the onset of the vertigo? Has there been any trauma? Drugs: Has the patient taken any medications? Associated symptoms: Is there a hearing loss or tinnitus? Has there been nausea, vomiting, nystagmus, or a visual problem? Does the patient have headaches?

The physical examination should include a complete neurological evaluation, as well as a psychosocial evaluation.

Psychological	Dizziness may occur secondary to neurogenic mechanisms. A vasovagal response to severe shock or fright may result in vertigo and syncope.
Benign Paroxysmal Vertigo	The onset is between 1 and 4 years of age. The attacks are characterized by unsteadiness and fear. The child may describe a spinning sensation. There is no loss of consciousness.
Epidemic Vertigo (Acute Labyrinthitis)	Epidemic vertigo is characterized by the acute onset of dizziness, nausea, and vomiting. Other symptoms may include diplopia and nystagmus. The course is self-limited and resolves spontaneously in approximately 2 to 3 days.

Drugs	Acetazolamide, antihistamines, colistin, diazepam, gentamicin, griseofulvin, indomethacin, isoniazid, kanamycin, nalidixic acid, phenothiazines, polymyxin, salicylates, sulfonamides, thiazides, and trimethoprim.
Hypoglycemia	Dizziness, pallor, diaphoresis, tachypnea, tachycardia, weakness, tremors, and convulsion are symptoms associated with hypoglycemia.
Anemia/ Hypovolemia	Anemia and hypovolemia may cause vertigo owing to the decrease in cerebral perfusion. Orthostatic hypotension frequently occurs. Because of the hypotension, dizziness or syncope may occur upon arising from the supine position.
Other Causes of Vertigo	Hyperventilation syndrome, seizure disorder, cerebellar tumor, abscess, lesions, acoustic neuroma, mumps, Ramsay-Hunt syndrome, vertebrobasilar artery occlusion, heat stroke, allergy, vestibular neuritis, increased intracranial pressure, and head injury.

Cause of Vertigo	Age of Patient	Aura	Vomiting	Nausea	Diplopia	Nystagmus	History of Drugs/Medications	Pallor	Diaphoresis	Tachycardia	Tremors	Loss of Consciousness	Seizures	Orthostatic Hypotension
Psychogenic	0	0	2	3	0	0	0	3	4	3	1	2	0	2
Benign paroxysmal vertigo	4	0	2	2	0	2	0	2	1	1	0	0	0	0
Epidemic vertigo/acute labyrinthitis	0	0	3	3	0	4	4	1	1	1	2	0	0	0
Drugs	0	0	2	2	1	3	4	1	1	1	0	1	1	0
Hypoglycemia	0	0	1	1	0	0	4	1	3	1	3	2	2	0
Anemia	0	0	3	3	0	0	4	4	2	3	0	0	0	3
Hypovolemia	0	0	3	3	0	0	1	4	4	4	4	1	0	4

Vomiting

Vomiting may stem from a number of causes. Generally, abnormalities of the gastrointestinal tract are considered first. Infants and children, however, may manifest vomiting with any systemic illness, as well as with such localized disorders as otitis media.

As with many other symptoms in the pediatric patient, age is of the utmost importance in formulating a differential diagnosis of the cause of vomiting. Vomiting in the neonate carries different implications than vomiting in the infant, older child, and adolescent. Other signs and symptoms may be present that may point toward a specific diagnosis.

It is important to determine the color and character of the vomitus. Other questions to pursue are: Is there any relationship of the vomiting to feedings or meals? Is fever present? Does there appear to be pain? Is pain or discomfort relieved after vomiting? What are the feeding habits? What foods (or other substances) have been ingested? Is there associated drooling? What are the character, consistency, and frequency of the stool? Is the patient urinating? Has there been any trauma? Are there any CNS, respiratory, or cardiovascular symptoms? Has there been any weight loss?

Regurgitation (Gastroesophageal Reflex)	A small amount of regurgitation is common in newborns and infants. It usually occurs when burping immediately after feedings. The volume is small and the regurgitation is not forceful. The material regurgitated has a normal odor. Minimal regurgitation is not associated with pathology.
Improper Feeding Techniques	Regurgitation and vomiting may occur following too rapid feedings or feeding of large volumes in a short period of time. Abdominal dis-

Improper Feeding Techniques (cont'd)	tension may be present. Babies with vomiting from this cause are frequently colicky. A careful feeding history must be taken. The vomiting commonly occurs soon after feeding or may be delayed by up to 1 hour. The vomitus appears relatively unchanged, lacks curds, and is not malodorous.
Rumination	Simple rumination in the very young infant is not uncommon. Persistence of rumination later in infancy and childhood signifies serious psychological pathology. Failure to thrive may be striking. The child will frequently make voluntary swallowing or gagging movements prior to the regurgitation, and will commonly manually gag itself, forcing vomiting and regurgitation. The vomiting has no relationship to feeding. The material produced is curdled and malodorous. Characteristic behavior patterns must be determined, and a psychological evaluation is necessary.
Excessive Crying	Vomiting may occur following forceful and excessive crying, secondary to increased intra-abdominal pressure with gastroesophageal reflux.
Other Causes of Nonorganic Vomiting	Feeding of solids before a baby can chew, motion sickness, functional causes, excitement, anxiety, imitative behavior, and as an attention-seeking device.
Esophageal Incoordination (EI)	Esophageal incoordination (EI) reflects abnormal esophageal peristalsis. Food and fluid are forced superiorly and inferiorly in a "sloshing" motion within the esophagus. Recurrent vomiting and regurgitation occur. In more severe cases, symptoms of failure to thrive may predominate. A barium meal with fluoroscopy will show "to-and-fro" movement of the barium.

Swallowed Maternal Blood	Hemoglobin is irritating to the gastrointestinal tract and may cause vomiting and diarrhea. The Apt test (see chapter on Hematemesis) can be used to determine fetal from adult hemoglobin.
Atresia, Stenosis, and Webbing	Any portion of the gastrointestinal tract may be atretic or stenotic. Webs are most frequently found in the esophagus and duodenum. The clinical presentations vary with the portion of the bowel involved. Symptoms of bowel obstruction predominate if the stenosis, atresia, or web is below the pylorus and above the ileocecal valve. Vomiting is frequently bilious. Abdominal distention and infrequent stools usually occur. Failure to thrive, weight loss, dehydration, and shock may also occur. Atresia of the large bowel, rectum, and anus presents with infrequent or absent stool, abdominal distention, and vomiting. With atresia, stenosis, or webbing above the pylorus, vomiting is usually the most striking symptom. The abdomen may be flat and distention is less frequent. Failure to thrive and dehydration may occur. Upper and lower gastrointestinal (GI) series and endoscopy may be diagnostic. A ''double-bubble'' on flat plate usually indicates duodenal stenosis.
Other Causes of Bowel Obstruction	Meconium ileus, functional ileus, meconium plug syndrome, annular pancreas, vascular rings, tumor, and duplication.
Pyloric Stenosis (PS)	Pyloric stenosis (PS) more commonly occurs in males. The onset of vomiting is usually during the third week of life. The vomiting is initially a mild regurgitation that progresses frequently to projectile emesis. A small, olive-shaped mass may be palpable. The patient may present with severe dehydration and metabolic

Pyloric Stenosis (PS) (cont'd)	alkalosis. The diagnosis is made through an upper GI series.
Tracheo-esophageal Fistula (TEF)	There are five types of tracheoesophageal fistula (TEF).
Esophageal atresia with distal TEF	The most common has a proximal blind pouch and a distal tracheoesophageal communication. Infants with this type of fistula will regurgitate and vomit all feedings. Choking, coughing, and cyanosis frequently occur. Profuse drooling may be present and the abdomen may be distended. A flat plate of the abdomen will show air in the stomach and intestines. A nasogastric or orogastric tube should be inserted and plain films of the neck, chest, and abdomen repeated. If there is a proximal blind pouch, the tube will be seen coiled in the pouch. A small amount of dilute barium may be injected to confirm the diagnosis.
TEF without esophageal atresia	A second type of TEF is the "H-type." There is continuity of the esophagus but a fistulous tract connects the trachea and esophagus. Infants with this type of fistula may appear normal; the only clue to the diagnosis may be frequent pneumonia. Rapid instillation of a dilute radiopaque fluid into the midportion of the esophagus may show filling of the fistulous tract.
Esophageal atresia with proximal TEF	With atresia of the esophagus and proximal communication with the trachea, the newborn presents primarily with severe respiratory tract symptoms: coughing, choking, cyanosis, respiratory distress, and aspiration pneumonia. Plain films will show aspiration pneumonia and absence of air in the gastrointestinal tract.

Esophageal atresia without TEF	In infants with esophageal atresia and no tracheal communication, the symptoms and signs are similar to those in the proximal blind-pouch type of TEF. Infants without the tracheal communication, however, have scaphoid abdomens, and plain films show no air in the gastrointestinal tract.
Esophageal atresia with proximal and distal TEF	The symptoms of this type are similar to esophageal atresia with proximal TEF. In this type, however, there will be air visualized in the gastrointestinal tract.
	Other congenital anomalies may be present in children with TEF. Cardiac anomalies are the most common, and the cardiovascular system must therefore be thoroughly evaluated in all children with TEF.
Chalasia	Chalasia is the reflux of stomach contents into the esophagus, and will result in frequent regurgitation in the infant. Normal cardioesophageal sphincter tone does not develop until 1 month of age, and gastroesophageal reflux can be demonstrated in almost half of all normal newborn infants. If chalasia is severe, anemia, esophagitis, hematemesis, and failure to thrive may occur. The diagnosis is made by fluoroscopy, demonstrating reflux of contrast material from the stomach into the esophagus during respiration, or by applying pressure to the abdomen.
Achalasia	Achalasia results from hypertonicity of the lower esophagus secondary to decreased ganglia in the myenteric plexus. The lesion is rare in children under 5 years of age. The most striking symptom is dysphagia, and longstanding difficulty in swallowing food is common. Children with achalasia eat very slowly. There is frequently retrosternal chest pain that may

Achalasia (cont'd)	be relieved with vomiting or swallowing movements. Failure to thrive may occur, as well as anemia, weight loss, coughing, wheezing, and recurrent pneumonia. The diagnosis is made through a barium meal. The esophagus will be dilated above a small, constricted segment. Abnormal esophageal peristaltic patterns may be demonstrated.
Central Nervous System Infection	Meningitis may present with vomiting as the only symptom in the infant. There may be fever. Meningismus occurs in the older child. The vomiting may be secondary to increased intracranial pressure, and may signify subdural effusion, especially in cases of *Hemophilus influenzae* meningitis; however, vomiting in the infant may occur without subdural effusion or increased intracranial pressure, since parenteral infection, independent of the site, may cause vomiting. Intracranial abscess frequently presents with vomiting. Fever, focal neurological signs, headache, nausea, and seizures may be associated findings.
Systemic Infection (Sepsis)	In the infant, any systemic infection may present with vomiting as an associated symptom; gastrointestinal infection need not be present for vomiting to occur. Poor feeding, fever, lethargy, irritability, and diarrhea may also be associated with parenteral infection.
Intracranial Tumor and Intracranial Bleeding	In the absence of infection, focal neurological findings, convulsions, cranial asymmetry, and abnormal behavior associated with vomiting should alert the physician to the possibility of an intracranial neoplasm. Ataxia may be present if the tumor develops in the posterior fossa. In the infant, bulging of the anterior fontanelle may signify increased intracranial pressure. It

Intracranial Tumor and Intracranial Bleeding (cont'd)	is important to take serial head circumferences, since a rapid increase in circumference signifies intracranial pressure. The etiology of the increased pressure may be tumor, intraventricular bleeding, subdural bleeding, or congenital defect in the ventricular system. The vomiting may or may not be projectile. The history may reveal trauma (in the case of bleeding). The trauma may seem trivial. Computed tomography and radionuclide brain scan will frequently be diagnostic in the case of an intracranial space-occupying lesion. Infection must be ruled out, and spinal tap should be done with extreme caution if there is any question of increased intracranial pressure.
Gastroenteritis	Vomiting may be associated with any type of gastrointestinal infectious process. Inflammation of the enteric mucosa, either by direct invasion or enterotoxin production, can cause vomiting, usually of sudden onset. Fever may be present, and there may be diarrhea and poor feeding. The degree of prostration depends on the length of illness and type and severity of infection. The state of hydration must be evaluated.
	Gastroenteritis may be caused by any agent irritating to the bowel; infection need not be present. Accurate dietary history is important. It is also important to determine whether any other family member is ill.
Drugs and Poisons	Pica and accidental ingestion of drugs or poisons must be considered when a child presents with vomiting and there is no apparent etiology. The emesis may be from direct irritation to the GI tract, or may be central in origin. Other signs of intoxication may be present and

Drugs and Poisons (cont'd)	should be looked for; these include constricted or dilated pupils, diaphoresis, tachycardia, tachypnea, tremor or fasciculation, wheezing, hypotonia, and hypertonia. The oral and pharyngeal mucosa should be evaluated for the presence of burns or lesions. Drug screening should be done and lead levels should be determined. Flat plate of the abdomen may show an ingested foreign body or the speckling of paint-chip ingestion.
Ketotic Hypoglycemia	This is the most common cause of hypoglycemia in childhood. The onset is between 15 months and 5 years of age. Vomiting, pallor, vertigo, ataxia, syncope, diaphoresis, tachycardia, tachypnea, convulsion, or coma may be the presenting signs and symptoms. There is usually a history of fasting. The hypoglycemic episodes resolve spontaneously after 9 to 10 years of age.
Reye's Syndrome	The sudden onset of vomiting 1 to 3 weeks after an acute viral illness (e.g., varicella, influenza) and central nervous system symptoms (e.g., confusion, disorientation, seizures, coma) should alert the examiner to the possibility of Reye's syndrome.
Other Causes of Vomiting	Hiatus hernia, pylorospasm, kernicterus, phenylketonuria (PKU), galactosemia, aminoaciduria, electrolyte imbalance, hyperammonemia (metabolic abnormalities), adrenal cortical hyperplasia, uremia, urethral obstruction, congenital renal anomaly, pertussis, celiac disease, intussusception, appendicitis, otitis media, testicular torsion, hepatitis, and pancreatitis.

Cause of Vomiting	Age of Patient	Relation to Food	Fever	Pain	Toxic or Acutely Ill Looking	Diarrhea	Constipation	Infrequent Stools	History of Ingestion	Drooling	Decreased Urine Output	Weight Loss	CNS Symptoms	Respiratory Tract Symptoms	History of Trauma/Surgery
EI/GER	4	4	*	0	0	0	0	0	0	0	0	0	0	*	0
Improper feeding technique	4	4	0	1	0	0	0	0	0	0	*	3	0	0	0
Rumination	4	0	0	0	0	0	0	0	0	0	*	4	0	0	0
Swallowed blood	0	0	0	0	*	0	0	0	0	0	0	0	0	1	1
Atresia, stenosis, webs	3	4	*	1	2	0	0	4	0	4	4	4	0	3	0
Pyloric stenosis	4	3	0	1	0–4	0	0	0	0	0	2–4	3	0	0	0
Tracheoesophageal fistula	4	4	*	0	2	0	0	4	0	3	*	4	0	3	0
Chalasia	4	4	0	1	1	0	0	0	0	0	*	3	0	1	0
Achalasia	4	4	0	3	0	0	0	3	0	0	*	2	0	2	0
CNS infection	0	0	3	0	4	0	0	0	0	0	0	2	4	0	0
Sepsis	0	0	4	0	4	2	0	0	0	0	*	2	*	*	0
Tumor (intracranial)	0	0	0	0	4	0	0	0	0	0	0	3	4	0	*
Acute gastroenteritis	0	2	3	4	0–4	4	0	0	0	0	3	3	0	0	0
Drugs	0	0	0	0	3	0	0	0	4	0	0	0	2	1	0
Ketotic hypoglycemia	4	0	0	0	3	0	0	0	0	0	1–4	1	3	1	0

continued

Cause of Vomiting (cont'd)	FTT	Voluntary Swallowing Movements	Gagging	Malodorous Emesis	Mass	Scaphoid or Flat Abdomen	Distended Abdomen	Projectile	Dysphagia	Chest Pain	Pneumonia	Meningismus	Focal Neurological Signs	Bulging Fontanelle
EI/GER	2	0	0	0	0	4	0	1	1	1	2	1	0	0
Improper feeding technique	3	0	1	0	0	2	2	1	0	0	0	0	0	0
Rumination	3	4	4	4	0	4	0	1	0	0	0	0	0	0
Swallowed blood	0	0	1	1	0	4	0	0	0	0	0	0	0	0
Atresia, stenosis, webs	4	3	4	1	0	2	2	0	3	0	2	0	0	0
Pyloric stenosis	3	0	0	0	3	2	2	3	0	0	0	0	0	0
Tracheoesophageal fistula	4	0	4	0	0	2	2	0	2	0	3	0	0	0
Chalasia	1	0	4	0	0	4	0	0	1	1	0	0	0	0
Achalasia	2	3	3	0	0	4	0	2	3	3	1	0	0	0
CNS infection	0	0	0	0	0	4	0	2	0	0	0	4	3	3
Sepsis	1	0	0	0	0	1	3	1	0	0	*	*	*	*
Tumor (intracranial)	1	0	0	0	4	2	2	2	0	0	0	0	3	2
Acute gastroenteritis	0	0	0	0	0	2	2	0	0	0	0	0	0	0
Drugs	0	0	2	0	0	2	2	2	0	0	0	0	2	0
Ketotic hypoglycemia	1	0	0	0	0	4	0	0	0	0	0	0	0	0

Weakness

Weakness may be either subjective or objective, and a symptom or sign. It may be generalized or focal in location, and may involve one or many muscle groups.

It is important to determine from the history whether the weakness is of acute or chronic onset. Is the weakness generalized? Does it involve one side of the body or a single extremity? Does the weakness involve both lower extremities or upper extremities? Have there been any recent illnesses? Is the patient taking any medication? Are the patient's immunizations up to date? Has there been any trauma?

The physical examination should seek to determine whether the weakness is real or pretended and whether there are associated hypotonia, cranial nerve involvement, or focal neurological signs.

Disuse/Trauma	Extremities immobilized for a significant period of time will become weak from disuse. Splinting, secondary to pain, may also cause weakness. If the disuse is prolonged, atrophy may occur.
Hysteria	Symptoms of hysteria do not follow any specific pattern. Usually, anatomical relationships are not followed, and the diagnosis of hysteria is made because of inconsistencies in symptoms and normal anatomical and physiological relationships.
Myasthenia Gravis *Transient neonatal myasthenia gravis*	Infants with this condition are born of mothers with myasthenia gravis. There are hypotonia, weakness, ptosis, and poor respiratory effort.

Persistent neonatal myasthenia gravis	Symptoms of this disease are identical to those of transient neonatal myasthenia gravis, but there is no evidence of myasthenia in the mother. The disease does not resolve. The eyes are most severely affected.
Juvenile myasthenia gravis	Ptosis and diplopia are the most frequent presenting symptoms of this disease. The intercostal muscles are usually affected. Characteristically, the weakness increases after repetitive movements and resolves after rest. Exacerbation and worsening of ptosis will occur after sustained upward gaze. The Tensilon® test, as well as electromyographic (EMG) studies, are diagnostic.
Muscular Dystrophy	The symptoms of muscular dystrophy are usually not noticed until after 3 years of age; however, delayed motor development may be seen. Difficulty in stair-climbing and pseudohypertrophy of the calf muscles are common presenting signs. Shoulder-girdle weakness may cause the patient, when held in the axillae, to slip through the examiner's hands. Gowers' sign may be present. The creatine phosphokinase (CPK) test and muscle biopsy are diagnostic.
Intracranial Abscess or Tumor	Unilateral limb weakness may suggest an intracranial space-occupying lesion. Other focal neurological signs may be present. The onset may be acute or gradual.
Other Causes of Weakness	Hypotonic states, glycogen storage disease, amyotrophic lateral sclerosis (ALS), peroneal muscular atrophy, diastematomyelia, intramuscular injections, cauda equina tumor, dermatomyositis, poliomyelitis, Werdnig-Hoffmann disease.

Cause of Weakness	No Specifications	Isolated Portion of Extremity	Single Extremity	Upper Extremity	Lower Extremity	Generalized	Cranial Nerve Involvement	Focal Neurological Signs	Hypotonia	Ptosis	Diplopia	Increased Weakness with Activity	Decreased Weakness with Tension® Test	Pseudohypertrophy	Gowers' disease	Increased CPK Level
Trauma	4	3	3	3	3	3	2	2	0	2	2	0	0	0	0	1
Disuse	4	4	3	4	4	4	0	4	4	4	3	0	4	4	4	4
Myasthenia gravis	2	0	0	0	0	4	3	0	4	4	2	4	4	0	0	0
Muscular dystrophy	4	0	0	3	3	3	0	0	4	3	3	2	0	4	4	4
Intracranial abscess/tumor	0	2	2	2	2	0	3	3	0	2	2	0	0	0	0	0
Werdnig-Hoffmann disease	1	0	0	2	1	4	0	2	4	0	0	2	0	0	1	0
Poliomyelitis	1	0	3	3	3	3	3	3	4	2	2	0	0	0	0	3

Wheezing

Wheezing is a symptom caused by a narrowing of the smaller bronchi and bronchioles. In children, the statement that "all that wheezes is not asthma" holds true; there are many, varied etiologies. Wheezing must be differentiated from stridor, which is low in pitch and results from narrowing of the upper airway (suproglottis, glottis, subglottis and trachea).

The examiner can obtain from the history a great deal of information that may point to the cause of wheezing. Specific questions to be asked are: Have there been any prior episodes of wheezing? Is there a family history of wheezing? Was the child eating or playing with a toy prior to the onset of wheezing? Did the child appear sick prior to the onset of wheezing? Does the child have any allergies? Has the child been taking any medication? Is there a history of eczema? Was the onset of wheezing acute or insidious?

In the physical examination, the examiner should differentiate between inspiratory and expiratory wheezing. Other questions to be answered in the physical examination are: Is the chest symmetrical? Are the breath sounds bilaterally equal? Are the heart sounds displaced? Is there any evidence of heart failure? Is the child in mild, moderate, or severe distress? Is the child febrile?

Asthma	Asthma is an acute respiratory illness characterized by reversible bronchospasm, excessive, tenacious mucus production, and mucosal edema. The attacks are episodic. There is frequently a strong family history of asthma. The patient may admit to allergies. There may be associated eczema. The acute episode is of

Asthma (cont'd)	sudden onset. Respiratory distress will vary from mild to severe. Physical examination will reveal diffuse, bilateral expiratory wheezing and a prolonged expiratory phase of respiration. The chest may appear "barrelled." To breathe, the patient usually uses all accessory muscles of respiration, causing intracostal, subcostal, and suprasternal retractions. There may be nasal flaring. Depending on the severity, cyanosis may be present. Chest X-ray films may reveal bilateral air trapping. Oral or parenteral bronchodilating agents, such as epinephrine and theophylline derivatives, will rapidly alleviate the reversible bronchospastic component of asthma.
	In children less than 6 months of age, the diagnosis of asthma is questionable even in the presence of a response to bronchodilating agents. During the acute phase of asthma, the patient is tachypneic and the blood gases will initially reveal hypocapnea. As the degree of airway obstruction increases, the pCO_2 will rise and approach normal values. If the obstruction continues, the patient will become hypercapneic and hypoxic. When the degree of obstruction is severe, respiratory failure may ensue.
Bronchiolitis	This is an acute infectious disease, occurring, most frequently, in children less than 6 months of age. There are an acute onset of wheezing, tachypnea, and respiratory distress. As in asthma, there are varying degrees of distress, depending upon the severity of the infection and the degree of bronchiolar narrowing. The wheezing is diffuse, and there may be associated rales and ronchi. The chest may appear "barrelled," and air trapping may be seen on

Bronchiolitis (cont'd)	chest film. The etiology is most commonly viral. The child is usually febrile and may appear acutely ill. Cyanosis may be present. The family history may or may not reveal asthma. There may be a variable response to parenteral bronchodilating agents such as epinephrine.
Pneumonia	Wheezing is a frequent symptom of pneumonia in childhood. The etiology may be viral, bacterial, or fungal. The wheezing occurs secondary to airway edema and mucus production. An element of irritative bronchospasm may be present or absent. A chest X-ray film may or may not show an infiltrate. Since X-ray film changes characteristically occur between 2 and 4 days after the onset of the clinical signs or symptoms of pneumonia, the patient may clinically have the signs and symptoms of pneumonia, yet demonstrate a normal chest X-ray film. In neonates, infants, and children, the differentiation between a viral and a bacterial etiology for pneumonia is difficult. Blood cultures positive for bacteria suggest a bacterial etiology for the pneumonia.
Foreign Body	The aspiration of a foreign body frequently presents with wheezing as a primary symptom; however, if the foreign body is lodged in the upper airway, stridor is more common. When the foreign body is located in the lower airway, wheezing will predominate. There may be a history of a choking episode followed by respiratory distress. Physical examination may reveal varying degrees of respiratory distress. There may be asymmetrical expansion of the chest. Decreased breath sounds and unilateral wheezing may be present. The wheezing may be inspiratory, expiratory, or both. Chest X-ray films may reveal infiltration or consoli-

Foreign Body (cont'd)	dation confined to a specific segment or lobe of the lung. Inspiratory and expiratory chest films may define the diagnosis. On inspiration, both lungs usually appear equally expanded. On expiration, the hemithorax in which the foreign body is located will remain hyperexpanded. The unaffected hemithorax will respond normally during expiration and its volume will decrease. During expiration, there may be a mediastinal shift away from the side in which the foreign body is located. Bronchoscopy is usually diagnostic and therapeutic. In the case of a "missed foreign body" there may be signs and symptoms of recurrent pneumonia. This diagnosis should be suspected in a child with recurrent pneumonia with infiltration of the same lobe or segment in each episode.
Other Causes of Wheezing in Children	Enlarged mediastinal lymph nodes, tumors, laryngotracheobronchitis, congenital heart disease, vascular anomalies, such as pulmonary vascular slings, anaphylaxis, drugs, cystic fibrosis, and bronchopulmonary dysplasia.

Cause of Wheezing	Paroxysmal	Acutely Reversible	Family History	Fever	Eczema	Allergies	Acute Onset	Unilateral	Bilateral	Distress	Responds to Bronchodilators	Bilateral/Symmetrical Air Trapping on X-Ray Film	Unilateral Air Trapping	S$_4$ Heart Sound	History of Medications	Age of Patient
Asthma	4	4	4	1	2	4	4	0	4	4	4	4	0	0	2	0
Bronchiolitis	0	2	2	3	0	1	3	0	4	4	1	4	0	0	0	4
Pneumonia	0	0	0	4	0	0	1–4	3	2	3	0	1	0	0	0	0
Foreign body	3	4	0	0	0	0	4	3	1	2	1	1	4	0	0	3
Congestive heart failure	3	3	0	0	0	0	1–4	0	4	1–4	1	0	0	4	2–4	0
Anaphylaxis	0	4	1	0	0	3	4	0	4	2–4	2	0	0	1	4	0

Bibliography

Books

Allen, J.E., Gururaj, V.J., and Russo, R.N. (1977): *Practical Points in Pediatrics*. 2nd ed. New York Medical Examination Publishing Company, Flushing, New York.

Apley, J., and MacKeith, R. (1968): *The Child and His Symptoms: A Comprehensive Approach*. 2nd ed. F.A. Davis Company, Philadelphia.

Barnett, H.L., Blatman, S., Brunell, P.A., Friedman, S.B., and Seidel, H.L. (editors). (1978): *Principles of Pediatrics: Health Care of the Young*. 16th ed. McGraw-Hill Book Company, New York.

Brimblecombe, F., and Barltrop, D. (1978): *Children in Health and Disease*. Baillière Tindall, London.

Davison, W.C., and Levinthal, J.D. (1961): *The Complete Pediatrician: Practical, Diagnostic, Therapeutic and Preventive Pediatrics*. 8th ed., revised. Duke University Press, Durham, North Carolina.

Ewerbeck, H. (1980): *Differential Diagnosis in Pediatrics*. Springer-Verlag, New York.

Fomon, S.J. (1967): *Infant Nutrition*. 2nd ed. W.B. Saunders Company, Philadelphia.

Gellis, S.S., and Kagan, B.M. (1976): *Current Pediatric Therapy, Vol. 7*. W.B. Saunders Company, Philadelphia.

Gellis, S.S., and Kagan, B.M. (editors). (1982): *Current Pediatric Therapy, Vol. 10*. W.B. Saunders Company, Philadelphia.

Green, M. (1980): *Pediatric Diagnosis: Interpretation of Symptoms and Signs in Different Age Periods*. 3rd ed. W.B. Saunders Company, Philadelphia.

Green, M., and Haggerty, R.J. (1977): *Ambulatory Pediatrics: II. Personal Health Care of the Child in the Office*. W.B. Saunders Company, Philadelphia.

Green, M., and Richmond, J.B. (1962): *Pediatric Diagnosis: Interpretation of Signs and Symptoms in Different Age Periods*. 2nd ed. W.B. Saunders Company, Philadelphia.

Groff, D.B. (1975): *Handbook of Pediatric Surgical Emergencies: A Guide to Emergencies in Pediatric Surgery*. Medical Examination Publishing Company, Flushing, New York.

Hart, F.D. (editor). (1973): *French's Index of Differential Diagnosis*. 10th ed. Year Book Medical Publishers, Chicago.

Hoekelman, R.A. (editor). (1978): *Principles of Pediatrics: Health Care of the Young.* McGraw-Hill Book Company, New York.

Huffman, J.W. (1969): *The Gynecology of Childhood and Adolescence.* W.B. Saunders Company, Philadelphia.

Illingsworth, R.S. (1973): *Common Symptoms of Diseases in Children.* 4th ed. F.A. Davis Company, Philadelphia.

Kadushin, A., and Martin, J.A. (1981): *Child Abuse: An Interactional Event.* Columbia University Press, New York.

Krugman, S., and Ward, R. (1973): *Infectious Diseases of Children and Adults.* 5th ed. C.V. Mosby Company, St. Louis.

Lanzkowsky, P. (1980): *Pediatric Hematology-Oncology: A Treatise for the Clinician.* McGraw-Hill Book Company, New York.

Levine, M.D. (editor). (1983): *Developmental-Behavioral Pediatrics.* W.B. Saunders Company, Philadelphia.

Levy, H.B., Sheldon, S.H., and Sulayman, R.F. (1984): *Diagnosis and Management of the Hospitalized Child.* Raven Press, New York.

Lieberman, E. (1976): *Clinical Pediatric Nephrology.* J.B. Lippincott, Philadelphia.

McMillan, J.A., Nieburg, P.I., and Oski, F.A. (1977): *The Whole Pediatrician Catalog: A Compendium of Clues to Diagnosis and Management.* W.B. Saunders Company, Philadelphia.

Nelson, W.E., McKay, R.J., and Vaughan, V.C. (editors). (1975): *Textbook of Pediatrics.* 10th ed. W.B. Saunders Company, Philadelphia.

Newberger, E.H. (editor). (1982): *Child Abuse.* Little, Brown and Company, Boston.

Reece, R.M., and Chamberlain, J.W. (1974): *Manual of Emergency Pediatrics.* W.B. Saunders Company, Philadelphia.

Rendle-Short, J., and Gray, O.P. (1967): *A Synopsis of Children's Diseases.* 4th ed. Williams and Wilkins Company, Baltimore.

Roy, C.C., Silverman, A., and Cozzetto, F. (1975): *Pediatric Clinical Gastroenterology.* 2nd ed. C.V. Mosby Company, St. Louis.

Royer, P., Habib, R., Mathieu, H., and Broyer, M. (1974): *Pediatric Nephrology.* Vol. XI. W.B. Saunders Company, Philadelphia.

Rudolph, A.M. (editor). (1982): *Pediatrics.* Appleton-Century-Crofts, Norwalk, Connecticut.

Smith, C.H. (1972): *Blood Diseases of Infancy and Childhood.* 3rd ed. C.V. Mosby Company, St. Louis.

Top, F.H. Jr., and Wehrle, P.F. (editors). (1976): *Communicable Infectious Diseases.* 8th ed. C.V. Mosby Company, St. Louis.

Tunnessen, W.W. (1983): *Signs and Symptoms in Pediatrics.* J.B. Lippincott, Philadelphia.

Wasserman, E., and Gromisch, D.S. (1976): *Pediatrics: A Problem Ori-*

ented Approach. Medical Examination Publishing Company. Flushing, New York.

Winters, R.W. (editor). (1973): *The Body Fluids in Pediatrics: Medical, Surgical and Neonatal Disorders of Acid-Base Status, Hydration and Oxygenation.* Little, Brown and Company, Boston.

Journals

Coleman, A.B., and Alpert, J.J. (editors). (1970): *The Pediatric Clinics of North America: Symposium on Poisoning in Children.* Vol. 17, No. 3. W.B. Saunders Company, Philadelphia.

Grand, R.J., and Watkins, J.B. (editors). (1975): *The Pediatric Clinics of North America: Symposium on Gastrointestinal and Liver Disease.* Vol. 22, No. 4. W.B. Saunders Company, Philadelphia.

Grosfeld, J.L. (editor). (1975): *The Pediatric Clinics of North America: Symposium on Childhood Trauma.* Vol. 22, No. 2. W.B. Saunders Company, Philadelphia.

Keitel, H.G., and Hammond, K. (editors). (1965): *The Pediatric Clinics of North America: Symposium on Pitfalls in Clinical Practice: II.* Vol. 12, No. 2. W.B. Saunders Company, Philadelphia.

Publications

Handbook of Common Poisonings in Children. (1976): DHEW Publication No. (FDA) 76-7004.

Subject Index

188